THE JUICE MASTER'S
Slim 4 Life

THE JUICE MASTER'S
Slim 4 Life
FREEDOM FROM THE FOOD TRAP

Jason Vale

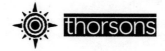

Thorsons
An Imprint of HarperCollins*Publishers*
77–85 Fulham Palace Road,
Hammersmith, London W6 8JB

The website address is:
www.thorsonselement.com

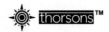

and *Thorsons* are trademarks of
HarperCollins*Publishers* Ltd

First published by Thorsons 2002

11

© Jason Vale 2002

Jason Vale asserts the moral right to be
identified as the author of this work

A catalogue record of this book is available
from the British Library

ISBN-13 978-0-00-713303-1
ISBN-10 0-00-713303-0

Printed and bound in Great Britain by
Creative Print and Design Wales, Ebbw Vale

Contents

1 Oh no! Not another diet book! 1

2 Never go on a diet again 8

3 Change your brand 22

4 We don't need to know 29

5 Why *do* people eat junk food? 35

6 Let's get physical 45

7 Oh sugar! 52

8 Fat free 58

9 Pinch of salt 64

10 The wonderful pleasures of eating rubbish 69

11 Change your mood by eating some food 77

12 Chocs away! 86

13 Out to lunch 92

14 Fast food 95

15 A meaty problem 101

16 'Dairy'-arians 110

17 Pasta la vista baby 118

18 Lethal combination 124

19 Con-appetite 130

20 Liquid asset 139

21 Diet Coke break 147

22 Coffee wake up call 152

23 Blind drunk 158

24 Pounds and pounds 169

25 The mouse trap 173

26 What you are giving up 180

27 The 'diet' recipe 184

28 The ultimate fat-busting health pill 199

29 The fastest food in the West 205

30 Furniture disease 213

31 The best exercise programme in the world 219

32 People phobia 224

33 Get busy living or get busy dying 234

34 The food police 240

35 Give your brain a break 245

36 Breakfast like a king 251

37 Let's do lunch 259

38 Go and play 263

39 What's for dinner? 264

40 Be flexible 267

41 You've got a ticket to the big game 271

42 Re-tune, re-tune and re-tune 275

43 JM's combining tips 280

44 Equipment 283

45 Recipes 287

46 Q & A 296

The Juice Master's page 309

1

Oh No!
Not Another
Diet Book!

That's right – what you are holding is *not* another diet book. In fact, if you're looking for something that is the complete opposite to the misery, deprivation and ultimate failure of dieting – then this is it.

This book is not just for people who are overweight either, it's for anyone who eats food – which pretty much covers everyone I think. And it's also not what I call a 'state the obvious' book either. What I mean is, I'm not going to spend the time we have together stating the mind-blowingly obvious to you about certain foods or treating you like some kind of idiot. That was one of the things I hated about eating the wrong foods, being overweight, feeling tired, lethargic and unhealthy myself – people assuming that just because I was thick physically, it automatically made me thick mentally. My doctor at the time was one of the worst for this and was head of what I call 'The State The Bleeding Obvious Brigade'. He would say things like, 'You're eating too much of the wrong types of foods, you don't exercise enough and you should lose weight. If you changed your eating habits and exercised more you would feel better and be slimmer.'

Well no shit Sherlock – you don't say! It was the same when I used to smoke 40–60 cigarettes a day; my doctor would say, 'It's killing you and costing you a fortune, you'd be richer and healthier if you quit.'

Once again – no really, hadn't figured that one out either doc. Now that you've told me I'll surely stop.

Doctors are not the only members of the 'State The Obvious Brigade' either; it appears most health books, diet clubs and people in general are also life-long members of it. What they fail to realize is WE ARE NOT STUPID. We know that things like chocolate, cola, coffee, cakes, crisps, ice cream, alcohol, milkshakes, and things like fast-food burgers and fries are not good for us and make us tired, ill and fat. We are also aware that fruit, vegetables, nuts, seeds, grains, fish etc. are all good and would keep us slim and healthy. I'm not being funny but who on earth doesn't know this? But does just knowing this help you to actually quit the unhealthy foods and change your eating habits in favour of the good stuff? No! If it did you wouldn't be reading this book, you would have already done it. And that's the problem. The instinctive knowledge that these foods are bad might make you think more about how much of them you are eating and thus make you try to control your intake of them on a consistent basis, but it doesn't stop you *wanting* them or having them. It certainly didn't stop me.

That is why I was always at least 30lb overweight, badly asthmatic, covered from head to toe in a skin disorder called psoriasis and had all the energy of a comatose dormouse. The only reason I didn't get even bigger was because I was *always* on a diet. The yo-yo king, that was me – always fighting a constant battle not to eat too much of the wrong kinds of foods; always using a degree of willpower, discipline and control to keep my health under some kind of control; always doing spats of 'healthy eating' and exercise to 'keep the weight off'. I hated it every time and always rewarded myself at the end of the nightmare with the very same stuff that caused the problem in the first place. I was more than fully aware that the foods I was eating were causing my physical problems – fat, lethargy and asthma – but the truth was I was *mentally* hooked at the time and simply didn't know what to do to escape.

So, if you thought you'd picked up a health book that was simply going to tell you that you should eat more fresh fruit and veggies, drink their fine juices, do more exercise and cut out the crap from your diet, you are very much mistaken. The reason is…

You already know you should do this

I knew it and so too do the millions of people around the world who are desperate to change their eating habits. I knew for certain that if I ate a lot of fruit and veg, stopped eating so much junk and went down the gym every now and then that I would be slim and healthy. But again, you hardly need to be Einstein to work it out now do you? Everybody already knows this – it's part of the 'bleeding obvious'. I will repeat again, simply being told that certain foods are good and others are bad does not make us change our eating habits – in fact, it's about as effective as a fishing trip on the Dead Sea!

THE FOOD TRAP

What you need, therefore, is not a lecture on the obvious, which will get you nowhere, but a full understanding of what I call 'The Food Trap'. You don't need a book explaining why you *shouldn't* eat certain foods – because you know why you shouldn't and by now are probably completely fed up with people telling you why you shouldn't. You need a full explanation of why you eat the foods you eat and why you eat at times to try and feed an emotion. You need to know exactly how the physical reactions caused by certain foods affect the way you think – how they *cause* cravings and *additional* hungers. You need a full understanding of what a craving really is, why it comes about and exactly how it can be easily shattered in a millisecond. You need to know exactly what is happening, both physically and mentally, when you eat things like sugar, fat, cakes, chocolate, coffee, cola, diet drinks, dairy products, red meat, etc. You also need to know precisely how the 'food' industry uses clever advertising and product placement to lure you into buying what I describe as 'drug foods', yes DRUG FOODS. You need to know how these drug food and drink companies manipulate your mind on a conscious and subconscious level to get you, and keep you, hooked on their 'brand' of junkie food and drinks. You need to know that many of the things that we believe, and have been told, are very good for us, are in reality causing incredible harm. You need to know how to find the mental inspiration to start moving your body again just for the sheer fun of it and not for 'weight loss' or to get 'healthy'. You need to discover 'the best exercise programme in the world' and when you do, I can guarantee you will not only love it but be totally inspired by it. And that, my friends, is what this book is about – everything you ever needed to know about exactly *what* to do both physically *and* mentally in order to break free from the food trap for life.

And when I say free I mean really free: free to move; free to eat what you want when you want; free from restrictions; free to think for yourself; free to look at people eating junk foods without any desire to do what they are doing; free from having to eat rubbish and then wish you hadn't; free to never go on a diet again; free from having to exercise control over certain foods on a constant basis; free from having to use willpower; free to wear what you want; and totally free to live the rest of your life in a slim, sexy, vibrant and energy-driven body. And that kind of freedom feels just soooo good, I can tell you.

And it doesn't matter what you have tried in the past or what you have been through, anyone – and having dealt with thousands of people I do mean *anyone* – can find it easy and enjoyable to change what they eat and drink and be slim, healthy and vibrant for life. All you need is an open mind and the conviction to finish the entire book. Most people who buy books of this nature don't even finish them and then complain that it was 'something else that didn't work'. This book really is different from any other food book you've read and I am very, very excited to share this information with you, but the only way your food problem can be solved for life, the only way you can possibly know exactly how to think in order to be slim and healthy for the rest of your life is if you…

Finish the whole book

The other thing you need to do is dump the past. Many people carry unwanted failures with them through life, constantly telling themselves that they can't succeed today because of what happened yesterday, or last week, or even 20 years ago! This prevents them from moving forward. It really doesn't matter how many times you've tried to change what you eat, get healthy, lose weight or all three, it doesn't

mean that you *can't* do it – it just means you've gone about it in the
wrong way. What's needed is something different.

'If you always do what you've always done,
you'll always get what you've always got'

I don't know who originally said that but they were bang on. I call it…

THE FLY SYNDROME

Have you noticed how flies keep banging themselves against the same
pane of glass in a desperate attempt to get out? And they continue to
do it even when there is an opening just above them. Why don't they
just fly slightly higher and set themselves free? The answer is very
simple – they cannot see that there is an easy way out and believe that
what they are doing will eventually set them free. And this is exactly
the same for the overweight/unhealthy person who keeps going on
diets or special exercise programmes that they hate in order to be slim
and healthy. They simply cannot see that there is an easy alternative.
They honestly think that if they just keep doing the same thing for
long enough that this approach will eventually set them free. But, just
like the fly, simply doing the same thing over and over again will *not*
produce a different result and will not set them free. I know because I
did more or less the same thing over and over again expecting to get a
different result – madness!

The truth is all the determination in the world would not enable the
fly to break through the glass – it needs to change its approach.
Exactly the same goes for you. Whether you know it or not at this
stage, you are in 'The Food Trap' and you can do all the affirmations,
positive thinking and be as determined as you like, but it won't set you
free – as you've no doubt experienced in the past. You may get
slimmer and healthier at times using this approach but it won't stop
you wanting junkie foods and having to exercise constant control over
them. In other words, you will still be mentally locked in the food trap.
I used to think that if I was managing to exercise control over my
intake of certain foods it meant I was in control. I now see that if you

are having to exercise control on a consistent basis it means you are being controlled, and if you are *being* controlled you are not free. What you need is an easy escape route from the sinister and subtle food trap. The exciting news is you're reading it.

So sit back, relax, *open your mind*, read at least a chapter every day to keep it fresh, and enjoy the journey. I will first explain the nature of the food trap, the nature of drug-like foods and drinks, and exactly why we all get sucked in – then I will give you the easy escape route to mental and physical freedom. I call it The Ultimate Health Recipe. Once you fully understand it, you will not only find the journey to perfect weight, excellent health and a truly energy-driven, vibrant, sexy body easy and enjoyable but, more importantly, you will be able to make the change *permanent.*

The aim is for healthy eating, juicing, blending and physical movement to become a daily part of your life so that you would feel deprived if you were not allowed to do it. Eating well and feeling physically fantastic will become as automatic as brushing your teeth. I want to explain to you how to give yourself supreme health, pure energy and a slim body forever, without having to 'give up' anything or make any kind of sacrifice.

As long as you dump the past and read this book with an open mind, by the time you finish it you will understand something that very few do: that ideal weight, great health, pure raw energy and physical and mental vibrancy are easily – yes EASILY – accomplished. It may be hard to believe at this stage – especially if you've tried God knows how times in the past – but, again, it's time to stop being a fly and open your mind to the fact that it's more than possible when you approach it in the right way. The truth is it's feeling sluggish, living with excess fat and ill health and constantly either trying to control your food intake or bingeing that is hard work.

BACK TO FRONT

This is where most people have got it wrong, as I did for many years. We believe that health is hard work – that we will have to go through some degree of torture to achieve the body of our dreams. Many of us think that it's easier to eat junk foods and stay unfit rather than go through the tremendous amounts of willpower, discipline and dedication – not to mention pain and hard work – we believe are necessary to achieve good health. That's why we don't get excited and look forward to getting slim and healthy – we assume that we will have to suffer in some way. That is exactly what I used to believe too. I now realize that a life of junk food, being unfit, hating the way you look and feel on an ongoing basis, and lacking in confidence is not easier – and it's certainly nowhere near as enjoyable as feeling alive, clearheaded, healthy, physically and mentally vibrant, and loving the way you look and feel.

We have a lot to get through and a lot of subjects need to be covered in order for you to break free. I want you to feel fantastic and live a quality of life, health-wise, that many people simply dream of. This book really is a catalyst to you getting there. There will be points in the book where you will want to start, where you think you've read enough and that you 'get it', but please, please…

DO NOT ATTEMPT TO CHANGE YOUR EATING HABITS UNTIL YOU HAVE READ THE ENTIRE BOOK

Do not go off 'half cocked' – you need the correct 'mental juice', otherwise in no time at all you could very easily switch to what I call 'diet' mentality. You need a *full* understanding of all junkie foods and drinks first. Only then will the mental instructions that will guide you out of the food trap make sense and prevent you from having to use your willpower, or as I call it 'the diet recipe'. That way you will not just be free, but you will feel free from the start and love the journey. So – in case I haven't yet mentioned it enough – please finish the *entire* book if you want true freedom from the food trap without having to diet ever again. And whilst I'm on that subject let me explain why diets (in the long run) do not work, can never work, never will work, so that you can finally feel totally free to…

2

Never Go on a Diet Again

Let me ask you a question. If I told you I had discovered a way to lose weight and gain health, would you be interested? Well, perhaps. However, if I explained that the method involves months of physical and mental torture, that you would have to opt out of life on a regular basis and feel miserable and deprived for months, that it would make you irritable, and involves incredible amounts of willpower, discipline and control, and, oh yes, I nearly forgot the best bit –

The method has a 95 per cent failure rate

Would you still be interested in trying it? In fact, would you invest incredible amounts of time, energy and money in anything that guaranteed a 95 per cent failure rate? I would have thought nobody in their right mind would do such a thing, and that is exactly the problem – many people are not in their right (frame of) mind. That is why millions of highly intelligent people diet despite knowing that at the end of their 'hard work' and misery they have a 95 per cent chance it will all have been for nothing. A 95 per cent chance of failing; and they are even aware of this fact before they begin. I'm not knocking them either, for I am certainly in no position to do so. After all, I tried many,

many diets myself. When I look back, I wonder why? Did it not dawn on me after my second diet that this approach was not going to work? A definition of madness is to do the same thing over and over again and expect a different result. 'But I've tried several different diets' you say. But have you? I thought I had tried many different diets but are they ever really that different? They all involve feelings of sacrifice, misery and deprivation. They all involve varying degrees of control and willpower. They all make you feel guilty when you're eating and down when you're not. They nearly always fail. They make you gain more weight than you had to begin with (if you're on a weight-loss diet). This is not one specific diet that I'm talking about – it's all of them. All diets are shining examples of the fly syndrome.

Despite knowing this, we still think that the next diet will be 'it' and seem willing to try anything, no matter how ludicrous or life-threatening it may seem. Since the original F Plan diet (and we all know that the F doesn't stand for fibre) we have tried eating grapefruits before every meal on the 'grapefruit diet' and even reached (or perhaps retched would be a better word) for that delightful smelling and tasting cabbage soup first thing in the morning on 'the cabbage soup' diet. Then there's the oranges and Alpen diet (one I made up and did for two months), the 'wedding dress diet' (but what happens *after* the big day), the 'Champagne and caviar diet' (you don't lose any weight, but you're so plastered you don't actually care) and the 'egg diet' (which involved eating 18 eggs a day). Then, of course, there's the Hay diet, the 'nothing but protein diet' (where your breath smells like Satan's bottom and, if you stick to it, you end up with a large head on a twig-like body), the many calorie-counting diets, the Kensington diet, the 'see' food diet, the Eat Fat Grow Slim diet (where you had to drink oil before each meal), the 'sex diet' (yes there is one – best of a bad bunch I'd say, and more fun than eating cabbage soup). And let's not leave out things like the Cambridge diet and all the other 'nutritious' shakes that promise fast weight loss. You may lose some weight but you'll soon put it back on. Why? Because you can't live on so-called nutritious shakes for the rest of your life. But 'nutritious' shakes seem like a highly intelligent thing to do compared to, wait for it – the 'Fresh Air' diet. Yes, let me repeat that –

THE FRESH AIR DIET

I wish I was joking, but it is perfectly true. There is a woman in Australia who has allegedly 'lived' on fresh air for years. She is apparently 'allowed' biscuits sometimes and lemon water, oh, and the odd chocolate. She claims to eat the same amount of food in one month as the average person eats in a day. Now you have probably heard of vegetarians, well, she is commonly known as a breatharian – yes, you do read correctly, a breatharian! The scary thing is that this woman has followers, and not just one or two, but hundreds. The fact that it was reported that three of her 'followers' died does not seem to dissuade her or her remaining followers. This is obviously the ultimate DIE...T! But all these diets are not a 'patch' on this crazy idea.

THE ULTIMATE WEIGHT LOSS PATCH

Someone has come up with the idea that if you are overweight the cause of your problem is you're low on patches. The Weight Loss Patch supposedly 'helps to melt away fat'. The theory is that if you shove loads of iodine into your bloodstream via a slow release patch you'll lose weight. Does it work? What do you think? Besides which, if this, or any product, did have the ability to increase the metabolic rate (which is what the iodine is supposed to do) it would have to be licensed as a drug and therefore wouldn't be available as an off-the-shelf slimming aid.

Then you have the Vanilla Patch, which is said to put you off eating chocolate. What you do is wear the patch on your hand and every time you feel the urge to have some chocolate you have a good sniff. I tried a similar thing when I used to smoke. I wore some patches to try and kick the habit – the problem was they contained the very same drug I was trying to kick, plus they were very difficult to light! From what I can see the only way these weight loss patches could possibly help you lose weight is if you stick them over your mouth.

The Vanilla Patch is not the only 'smelling' aid designed to help you lose weight, let's not forget Aromatrim (from the US – where else?). These patches are a nasty-smelling blend of ingredients that, according to users, smell 'like sweaty socks'. What you are meant to do if you feel like, say, some chocolate, is to take a good sniff of your Aromatrim and your craving will vanish. Does it work? Well it's spooky because their research says yes it does and yet my research (i.e. most of the people in the real world I know who have tried it) says NO IT CLEARLY DOES NOT. One of their marketing directors, Carol Fountain, says, 'It has been tested successfully on thousands of Americans'. But what the hell does *tested successfully* mean? It could just mean that the company has been *successful* in getting people to test it, but does that mean for one second that the people who tested it were successful in ending their cravings for good?

Never mind though, because if all these diets and patches fail you can always try Speed – oh sorry, I mean 'slimming pills'. This is where you lose weight by whizzing around like a deranged blue-arsed fly doing mad things like hoovering the house at 3am because you've falsely stimulated your nervous system so much you can't sleep.

But why do we try any of this nonsense? Most of us, to be fair, skip the patches and smelling nonsense but diets, why do we do it? Why do we go on *any* specialized diet? Do we not already know what to do in order to lose weight and gain health? Could you not write down at least ten different ways to lose weight that – if you followed them – would all work? Could you not also design yourself an exercise programme that – if you followed it – would make you lean and fit? I think that we are intelligent enough to realize that if we ate nothing but cabbage for three weeks we would lose weight (and most of our friends too) and that if we ate loads of fruit and veg and drank their juices we would be very, very healthy. I knew exactly what to do to lose weight and gain health, but I did not know how to do it and more importantly how to *enjoy* the process at the same time. Nor did I know what to do to make it permanent – the most important part.

TELL ME WHY I DON'T LIKE MONDAYS

When I started any of my diets I would immediately suffer, not physically but mentally. I would always start my diet on Monday (when else?). If people just stopped going on a diet they would instantly eat less junk anyway. When I knew I was going on a diet on Monday, I would eat as much rubbish as I possibly could from the Friday onwards declaring 'It's okay, I'm going on a diet on Monday'. So I would always eat a lot more than I would have normally eaten if I hadn't made the conscious decision to 'diet'. Half way through Tuesday and the inevitable 'I've picked the wrong time' would rear its ugly head. This would be rapidly followed by 'The bomb could go off tomorrow' and 'What's the point of living?' and I'd be back where I started. Well not quite – usually I'd then eat more than normal to subconsciously make up for lost eating time.

On other occasions I would not call it a 'diet' but simply say 'As from Monday, I will start to eat healthily'. Now I am sure that whoever invented the fridge hated fruit and veg. There is that drawer at the bottom to put your veg in so that you can conveniently forget that it's there – only to re-discover it days later when it's beginning to make its own way out! You then throw the mouldy veg in the bin with the declaration, 'I forgot all about that, if I'd have remembered I would have eaten it. Oh well, let's go get a take-out – it doesn't matter because I've decided to make a fresh start...on Monday.'

I never got excited about getting a slim physique and gaining health because of the awful trauma I *thought* I had to go through in order to achieve my goal. I now realize the real trauma was to do with having the junk, not doing without it. But if you are psychologically hooked on 'foods' that you know are causing you problems; if you believe that you actually gain something from them – whether it be pleasure, comfort or whatever – then those foods do not become less precious if you are forced to do without them. As you have no doubt experienced, they become the most precious thing in the world. Your entire focus is on either eating them or not eating them – as a result you experience the mental trauma that so many people go through.

When I was on a diet I would 'hang on in there' for as long as I could, trying to stop myself from consuming the foods that I *thought* I wanted; foods I genuinely believed would benefit me in some way, even if the benefit was only momentary. The problem with this is there is only so long that anyone can 'hang on in there' for. No wonder I never succeeded on a diet. No wonder it has such a high failure rate.

And that is the real problem with diets – you force yourself to do something which you do not want to do in the hope that you will reach what you do want i.e. your ideal weight or optimum health. But all the time you are doing something you don't want to do you are effectively having an internal, and often external, tantrum. One side of your brain wants the junk but the other half doesn't because you want to look and feel better: 'Yes I will, no I won't' – it's a constant mental battle. There is only so long you can do this before you say 'Sod it!'

At what point do we ever feel free from this mental battle? I use the term 'free' to describe not having to worry about the food we eat or having to exercise discipline and control over our intake; I mean truly free to eat, free from guilt. So when are we free? The minute the diet is over? NO. Because we then start to eat the same junk again and the battle starts all over again. And, of course, every time we diet we end up with a *bigger* battle on our hands, both physically and mentally. When you have been knocked down just once it's easy to pick yourself up. If you keep getting knocked down you end up thinking 'what's the point in getting back up?'

The answer is to remove the very thing that is knocking you down – this is not simply the food itself, but the conditioning, brainwashing and misinformation that is the *cause* of why we put this stuff in our mouths. All these factors encourage the belief that life would not be as enjoyable without junk and drug-like foods; that life would be 'dull' and 'boring' if we ate healthily and did exercise; that people who do this are boring, no-hope health freaks who have forgotten how to live; that it is a 'constant battle' to be healthy and maintain your ideal weight. I used to believe this rubbish too.

Two of the main weight loss clubs in the world also perpetuate the belief that it's a lifetime battle – so much so that you have to attend their meetings every week just to make sure you are still on track, that you haven't 'fallen off the food wagon'. Yes I am talking about Weight Watchers and Slimming World. Now, before I go on, I must say that I am fully aware that both of these organizations have helped many, many people throughout the world. But however admirable their motives might be, they are instilling in the person with a 'food problem' the notion that they will have to try and 'control' their weight forever and it will be a constant battle. Not only must they come back week in week out, but they must follow a system of counting 'points' or 'sins'. At Weight Watchers you get extra points if you do a certain amount of exercise. And what do points make? Food. People end up exercising simply so that they can have some cake!

TOTALLY POINTLESS

The Weight Watchers points system is by no means a new concept for restricting food intake either. Did you know that as far back as the late '30s and early '40s there was a very similar points system used for restricting people's intake of food? It was called the 'Rationing' club! Yes, when food was scarce in the war people were given ration books and were allocated what were literally called 'Personal Points' for each day. You were allocated a certain amount of points and each food had a 'value' – sound familiar? The big difference was, no one was in the rationing club voluntarily and no one was pleased to be losing weight either. The whole business of counting the 'points' value of certain foods and rationing yourself accordingly is nothing short of madness. I bet there was not one single person in the war who ever thought they would see the day when people would actually pay for the privilege of *deliberately* restricting the amount of food they were allowed by counting 'points' – especially in times when food is in abundance!

The diet clubs give the impression that if you don't count points and attend weekly meetings that you will binge and go back to your old 'habits'. Overeaters Anonymous (yes there is such an organization) take the idea of the 'constant battle' even further by suggesting that the 'problem' is due to some kind of weakness inherent in you, rather than with the drug-like foods themselves. OA has a twelve step plan to help you 'cope with' your disease. Yep! that's what they call your problem – a disease. The twelve step plan is to help you cope with, not cure, your disease. For as far as they are concerned the disease is caused by something in your genes and there is no known cure. You were born with it and there is nothing you can do about it. How's that for setting yourself up for failure? That to me is the same as seeing someone sinking in quicksand and saying that the reason they're sinking is nothing to do with the quicksand – they were born with a quicksand sinking gene.

Sadly, it seems we are willing to take advice from virtually anyone – regardless of whether or not they are ill and fat themselves. Many of the 'leaders' running the 12,000 slimming clubs in the UK are often 'yo-yoing' themselves – still constantly having a battle with food, their health and their weight. Now if you went to a 'stop-smoking' therapist to quit smoking and they had a cigarette hanging out of their mouth, would you listen to a word they have to say to you, even if the advice was correct? No way. Don't get me wrong, I'm not picking on these people (after all, I know what it's like to be in the food trap and it's really not that funny to be constantly struggling with your health, weight and food intake), I just don't think they should be teaching to others what they are clearly struggling with themselves.

The overall position of the 'diet' industry seems pretty clear then. When it comes to weight loss and changing eating habits we have only two choices: either exercise control forever, or run out of the will to control, say 'sod it' and binge – then after the binge go back to trying to control again for a while. What a life! It seems to be a no-win situation – miserable when you are allowed to eat the junk and miserable when you're not. The good news is that there *is* an alternative and, as I have said, you are reading it. The best part of all is that when you see it clearly, when you know how the brain works and are in the right frame of mind, the whole thing becomes a piece of cake (figuratively speaking of course).

The diet mentality doesn't just apply to people who are overweight. There are many slim people who want to change their diet because they want to feel fitter and healthier and have more energy. But they too have the same problem. They want to be healthy, but they also want to eat junk. So they have to force themselves to do something which they do not want to do in order to reach their goal. They too believe life would be nowhere near as enjoyable if they ate healthily.

In reality, one of the main reasons for this belief are the diets themselves. They encourage us to believe that life is awful without junk food, simply because we are so bloody miserable when we're on a diet and trying to resist it! Obviously when we are *not* on a diet we are slightly less miserable than when we are on one; but we are still miserable. That is why we want to change. It doesn't seem to occur to us that even when we are not on a diet we are still more miserable than someone who doesn't have to worry about their intake of food, their health or their weight. It wasn't only when I was consciously on a diet that I had this 'I want junk, but I wish I didn't' mental tug of war. The truth is I always had it to some degree. I was constantly trying to control my intake of food. On a diet I just had to try and control it even more than usual – which made me much more aware of it.

It is having to exercise control over your intake of food on a daily basis that is the problem. You shouldn't have to control what you eat, you should be free to eat whatever you want, whenever you want, without having to worry about your health and weight – just like *all* wild animals on this planet. Non-smokers can smoke whenever they want – they just don't want to so there is no problem. It is only smokers that have the problem of trying to control their intake, non-smokers have their freedom – the freedom of not having to smoke. I can eat junkie food whenever I want, but I just don't want to. It is only those people who are psychologically hooked on junk that constantly have to try and control their intake to varying degrees. Non junk-food eaters have their freedom – the freedom of not having to eat junk.

Wild animals have this freedom too. In fact we are the only creatures on the planet that do this control and dieting stuff. You don't ever see a squirrel weighing its nuts do you (bad analogy, I know)? Why not? Because they don't have television, radio and so-called 'experts' telling them what to eat or when to eat. They rely on their natural instincts. We also instinctively know exactly what to eat and when to eat. Our problem is that we have an intellectual brain that can easily be 'washed' by people with all kinds of vested interests. However, if we were left to our own devices we would all be eating healthily and no one would have a 'food problem'.

DIETS STARVE THE BODY AND MAKE YOU FATTER

Dieting itself creates food problems, it doesn't solve them. Diets never get rid of your food problem – they make it worse. You are no longer allowed to eat the 'brand of food' that you normally eat (your favourite foods). So even if you do stick to a diet and reach your goal, what happens when the diet is over? You 'reward' yourself – with what? Your favourite foods; after all you deserve a 'treat' for all the effort you have put in. You feel 'good' for such a short time because you soon realize you are getting unhealthy or gaining weight again. Once this starts to dawn on you, you either give in to it, or exercise control over your intake once again. The point is that you are never truly free. All you have in fact 'treated' yourself to are feelings of guilt, self-loathing, lethargy, a body you hate, and a life-time trying to control the cravings for your favorite foods. And how do we try and solve that problem – a diet!

Another major problem with diets is that you literally starve your body when you go on one (even more so than you do normally – I will explain later how most people are slowly starving themselves any-way). If you deliberately stop yourself eating when your body is screaming for food, you are fighting against the most powerful instinct in the world: survival. No wonder people find it hard. When you do this your body's metabolism slows down; yes *down*. If it keeps going at the rate it is with this little food coming in, you will die very quickly. So the minute the body senses that there is a severe lack of food coming in, it assumes you have no choice. And rather than let you die, your metabolism slows down considerably to conserve energy. At the same time, the body stores even more of what you do eat as fat as it senses lean times ahead. Because the fat is needed, the body even begins to burn muscle tissue, which is a bit of a bugger as muscle helps to burn excess fat – so double whammy! In fact, virtually every time you go on a restrictive diet you lose muscle tissue and gain more fat cells.

MORE PROBLEMS

When you start to eat 'normally' again (after you either say 'sod the diet' or you somehow manage to reach your physical goal) your metabolism is still working *slowly*. It will not increase until it knows for sure there will be enough food coming in on a regular basis. This can take weeks or even months. The body also wants to make sure it has enough fat in reserve in case it happens again and so is loath to let go so quickly.

So, having acquired a slower metabolism, you now go back to eating exactly the same amount of food you ate before you started the diet. And what happens? You put on *more weight* than before you started the diet – and, it seems, a lot faster than it took to shift it. This is not simply your perception either. A study carried out on a group of rats in 1986 showed that by the time they did their second diet, the weight loss was half of what it was the first time and, wait for it, the weight was put back on THREE TIMES AS FAST. This is happening to millions of people around the world as we speak. The problem is it's a cause and effect chain reaction, for when you see the weight rapidly piling on again you once again think that it's time to do something about it – what? Oh yes the latest DIET.

So what's the choice? Well if you give your metabolism some time it will eventually stabilize and increase by the amount that was lost because of the diet. Most people do not know this (as I didn't for years) so their 'food problem' always gets that little bit worse. Now I understand why dieting makes people fat. It helps create the problem they are trying to solve. It is only in fairly recent times that people have reached over 500lb in weight. If you keep going on a diet the body will hang on to more and more reserves for longer in case it happens again, and it will be loath to let it go if food stops coming in again. This cycle helps to keep people unhealthy and fat.

Physically and psychologically diets are a complete nightmare. You never break free from the constant mental battle of trying to control your favorite foods, or the many physical problems they create – all that happens is you become totally obsessed with food. In short, diets mess you up big time. If you get nothing else from this book do yourself one of the biggest favours of your life and –

Never go on a diet again

Doing that alone will improve the length and definitely the quality of your life. If diets worked there would be one diet. As it is there are over 300,000 'different' diets to choose from, with plenty more on the way.

Some people are so desperate to get rid of their excess weight that they resort to the surgeon's knife. They cut out dieting in the hope they can literally cut out the fat with a knife or suck it out with a vacuum. Once again this only treats the *physical* side of the problem – usually not very well and sometimes with horrific results. What chance do people have of getting slim and healthy for *life* by simply cutting open the body and trying to carve out the excess fat – whilst still eating and drinking the same rubbish? Slim and none.

BAND AID

There are all kinds of ops out there to treat 'fat' – many of them costing thousands of pounds. One operation people can have is the 'gastric lap band'. This little beauty is like one of those jubilee clips, you know, the metal clips that are used to put pipes on taps etc. The difference is these are not made of metal and are not used to tighten up pipes – they are used to tighten up the stomach. They put an adjustable band around the top half of the stomach so you can only eat smaller portions. There is, however, a slight flaw in the plan – IT DOES NOTHING TO STOP YOUR MENTAL CRAVINGS OR INTAKE OF THE SUBSTANCES THAT CAUSE WEIGHT GAIN. You can still eat loads of sugar and fats – as long as you chew them enough and they are in more or less a liquid form, they can still pass through.

This is why one lady lost just 1lb in the seven weeks following this op. She spent £6000, went through the nightmare of being under the surgeon's knife to have her stomach strangled, yet still has *exactly* the same problem as before. She still battles every day with the mental cravings she has for the chocolates, cola, cakes, and all the other artificial sweet things that are causing the problem – and she still eats them. She is still on a permanent mental diet – still constantly trying to fight a desire to eat and drink certain foods. And exactly the same can happen with stomach stapling, jaw wiring, the stomach 'pace-maker' (yes there is one) or any of the other drastic surgical methods used to try and shift the fat.

THE FAT PILLS

But if the surgeon's knife is not your thing, then let's not forget that
the good old pharmaceutical companies are more than willing to help
you with their magnificent array of anti-fat pills. Yes, when all else
fails, give them a pill – that's the answer. Not all these pills are made
by the pharmaceutical industry: it seems anyone is allowed to throw a
few ingredients together, grind them into a powder, shove them into
a pill, give it a 'slimming' name and watch the pounds roll in. We have
everything from 'Fat Magnets', which claim to 'trap the fat before it's
absorbed into the bloodstream', to things like Xenical, Diet System 6,
Chrome Plus, Bran Slim, Figure Trim 8 and God knows how many
more. Xenical is one 'slimming' pill that is produced by one of the
huge pharmaceutical giants and you do need a prescription for this
little beauty. They claim that 30 per cent of the fat eaten in a meal gets
passed through the gut undigested with the 'help' of Xenical. 'So
what's the problem?' you ask, 'they sound ideal'. Ummmm, here's the
problem – they cause anal leakage. Yes, just when you least expect it –
BOOM! The undigested fat comes creeping out of your anus – without
warning. Beautiful. It is also said to cause foul-smelling stools and
stomach problems. Even the manufacturer's research showed that
only 1 in 4 cases showed any benefit and the benefit was only an extra
4 kilos of weight loss compared to diet alone.

The main problem with all these diet pills is that they once again do
nothing to deal with the cause of the problem: how you *think* about
food – your mental cravings. They also give people a false sense of
security so they tend to eat more anyway thinking, 'it's okay because
my Fat Magnets or whatever will deal with it'. These fat pills also
perpetuate the huge myth that it's the fat you eat that makes you fat.
As you will read later, this is total rubbish. In addition, they promote
the extremely damaging idea that any fat on the body is bad. It's all
about getting abnormally supermodel 'thin' as quickly as possible – no
matter what the cost. Ironically the cost is always *more* weight, an
unhealthy body and another foot further down in the food trap.
Talking of 'thin', one of the most dangerous diet fads to catch on, one
which totally focuses on the 'thin' and sod the healthy, is the…

EAT NOTHING BUT PROTEIN DIET

Will you lose weight eating nothing but protein? Yes. Is it healthy? NO IT IS NOT. Will it last for life? Like any diet, what do you think? Even the late Dr Atkins, who became infamous for his high-protein regime, was reported to be overweight himself! This is not a way to get slim and healthy for life – it's a way to get unnaturally thin whilst beating up your organs, speeding up the ageing process, smelling like the breath monster and, oh yes, going insane – all at the same time. Oh and then ultimately failing anyway. The people who promote the high protein, high fat diet even suggest eating fried eggs and bacon in the morning and claim it's healthier than eating fruit! The problem is many of the people who follow it have been so sucked in by the babble that they believe it too.

The point is, are any of these so-called solutions, whether it be diet, patch, pill, or surgeon's knife, going to solve your problem for life? NO WAY. All they do is put you through mental and physical discomfort in order to be temporarily slim. And what the hell do they do for your health and longevity? SOD ALL. All they do is treat the *physical* symptoms of being mentally locked into the food trap, but they do nothing to set you truly free.

'Okay,' you say, 'I now realize that dieting is a waste of time and effort, that pills only exasperate the problem and that surgery is a complete nightmare, but what is the alternative? If I want to get healthy, have more energy and lose weight then surely I will still have to discipline myself not to eat my 'favourite foods'? So how can I ever be free?'

The good news is, as I promised at the start of the book, it's very easy to have ideal weight and optimum health. It's very easy to get rid of your 'food problem' for life and have true freedom. The answer is not cutting down on your 'brand of food' or starving yourself, but simply changing the way you think about foods in order to successfully...

3

Change
Your Brand

When I was unhealthy, tired, lethargic and overweight, I knew that if I ate plenty of fruit, vegetables and salads I would be slim and healthy. But the problem was that I didn't like them and I didn't want to eat them. They were not my 'brand of food'. I had fruit every now and again – summer mainly – and even then only the odd orange. As for salads, somehow I don't think the token side salad, which I hardly touched, really counted. The main difficulty I had was that I simply didn't like the taste of vegetables and salads. And even the fruits I did eat didn't seem to satisfy me the same way as steak and chips. Besides which, I had always been conditioned to believe that if you ate that 'rabbit food' you were being boring. No, my brand of food was steak and chips, McDonalds, Burger King, chocolate, crisps, a big 'hearty' breakfast, tons of tea and coffee, bread and butter, big helpings of white pasta, egg or beans on toast, hot dogs, Sunday roast. In fact, you name it I ate it – as long as it wasn't green. I often looked at well-prepared, beautiful-looking salads and thought, I really wish I liked that, but I just don't. If I could get as much pleasure and satisfaction from eating fruit, salad, vegetables and drinking carrot juice as I do eating steak and chips and drinking Coke, then I would do it – who wouldn't?

The excellent news is that you can – easily. I know at this stage that may sound like rubbish or unbelievable, especially for those who have tried 'everything' in the past, but I did say at the start that an open mind is required for success. In reality not only will you get as much pleasure and satisfaction from your new brand, but infinitely more so. These days I wouldn't even let you pay me to eat steak and chips and I certainly would never, and I mean NEVER drink something like Coke. Yet for years these were my 'brands' of food and drink; in other words, my favourite foods.

When I wake up in the morning now and head straight for my juicer and blender, I do so not because I 'have to' or because I need to lose weight due to some restrictive diet. I do so because I now wouldn't dream of doing anything else – I choose to do it, I want to do it. I am writing this with some surprise because only a few years ago the first thing I 'had' to do was stick the kettle on to give myself a caffeine 'boost' in the morning. I now know this was to try and get me over my junk and drug food hangover (more about that later). I would then eat a big bowl of cereal, several rounds of toast and maybe a couple of boiled eggs. At the weekends my breakfast consisted of everything that was on offer at JJ's café. The great British breakfast – the bedrock of a good heart attack as they say.

I used to have images of people who owned a juicer, drank carrot juice and ate leaves. One which perhaps you have at the moment. I would think 'What sad and boring people, what on earth do they do for fun?' But who was I kidding? As if I was having fun being overweight, tired, lethargic, hating the way I felt and looked, constantly battling with my intake of food and my health, always battling with the latest new health 'diet'. And all for what? What was my trade off? What was I getting that was so brilliant? The wonderful pleasures of my favourite foods? I always thought that if I stopped eating the junk I would be making a sacrifice: if I drank fresh juice, ate good food, created the body I wanted, felt light, and had the energy to literally suck the juice from daily life, that I would somehow be missing out. But on what? When I ate a chocolate bar I would always think 'I wish I hadn't done that' or 'why did I do that'. I never really enjoyed the taste as it would be gone in seconds. I was setting myself up for a lifetime of misery, lethargy and being overweight all for literally seconds of what I thought was genuine pleasure – even though I hated myself the very second I ate it. Hardly a fair trade off now is it?

I often felt bloated after eating a pile of my 'favourite food'. My physical problems were clearly caused by my favourite foods. These foods would always seem nice in my mind before I ate them, but as soon as I did, I wished I hadn't. That's not satisfaction, it's the complete opposite.

What was so special about my old favourite foods? What did they do for me? Since changing my brand I now see the truth – there was nothing special about these foods. I now see they do nothing for you. And I do not simply mean the disadvantages outweigh the advantages, you know that already. What I mean is that there are no advantages in consuming junkie-type food and drinks on a consistent basis (as you will clearly see by the end of this book).

The superb news is that contrary to what we have been conditioned to believe it is very, very easy to switch 'brands' (change your diet in other words). I know many people who used to take sugar in their tea but now wouldn't pay you for a cup with even a grain in it. Why not? What has changed? The tea and the sugar have always remained exactly the same. The difference is they have simply trained themselves to *like* tea and coffee without sugar. The process is not hard, in fact it usually takes all of a week to get used to any new taste. The week is not painful just a bit strange at first, like any change. The coffee without sugar does not taste wonderful at first but after a while it tastes better than it did with sugar in. The point that I am making is that these people now would *never* drink tea or coffee with sugar in it again. Not because they *can't*, or because they are being forced not to, but because they have no *desire* to any more – they have changed their brand. Having done so they will *never* have to use willpower, discipline or control *not* to have sugar in their tea for one simple reason; it is now what they prefer – it is now their brand. This means their sugar problem has now been solved for life. They will never have to go on a 'no sugar in coffee diet' ever.

This is why it is so easy to have good health, energy, vibrancy, a slim physique and love the way you feel. The answer is not to diet, but simply change the way you think in order to change your brand. Unless you change your taste buds and how you view foods in your mind, you will *always* have a food problem.

If you change your brand (which takes all of a week, possibly two, to get used to) you never have to think about your health or weight and your 'food problem' will be gone forever. And once I give you all the instructions at the end, you will even *enjoy* the adjustment. Just imagine having no desire to eat rubbish, not envying the people who are eating it and genuinely relishing and loving the good stuff. When you finish this book and follow the Ultimate Health Recipe you won't have to imagine – it will become your reality.

I want to make this point clear: I am not being 'good' drinking 1–2 pints of freshly extracted juice daily and skipping the junkie food – no more than people who no longer take sugar in their tea are being 'good' for not putting sugar in. They simply have no *desire* to go back and I have no desire to go back. Are you being good for not taking heroin? Do you feel proud of yourself because you haven't sniffed glue today? If you did feel proud then it would mean that you indeed have a glue problem. I am not proud of myself for not eating junk today, I just don't want to eat this stuff as my main diet any more. Unlike a conventional diet (in the restrictive sense), I *can* have whatever I want now, I no longer have to put restrictions on myself. The difference is that I just do not want them any more. I am not being good for eating my new brand, I *want* to eat it (or drink it) – it is now my genuine choice. I am not continuing to do what I do to lose weight, because I'm already slim, and I'm not doing it to stay slim – I'm doing it because it is now my brand and I love it!

A few years back I would never have believed that I could literally train myself to love fruits, salads, vegetables and their juices. But, as macrobiotics has been teaching for years, you will adapt and learn to love any food or drink you have on a *regular* basis (I'm not sure Brussels sprouts are included in that mind you). That is something I would have dismissed in an instant a few years ago, but it's true. Years back I tried some Chinese herbal medicine in an attempt to clear my skin of psoriasis. The best way I can describe the medicine is tree bark – literally. I had to boil what looked like bits of tree and forest detritus in water twice every day. To say this stuff stank would be putting it mildly and it tasted as bitter as a winter's night in Halifax. I hated it to say the least, but I drank it as I was willing to try anything. As I drank this warm muddy-looking water, I would hold my nose and try not to be sick – it really was that bad. Here's my point: within one month, not only did I get used to the smell and taste – I actually began to like it. This is why changing your brand of food is going to be a breeze once we remove the brainwashing and I give you a set of easy mental instructions. After all, nothing you switch to will taste and smell anything like tree bark so the adjustment won't take anything like a month and you certainly won't be holding your nose and trying not to be sick during it. In fact, most of the things many of you will already love. But it really doesn't matter if at this stage a main course salad and some vegetable juice sounds about as appealing as a fortnight's holiday in Afghanistan. Once all the brainwashing, conditioning and misinformation regarding your current brand of foods and drinks has been removed, and you have the mental and physical instructions on exactly how to change your brand *easily*, you will be as amazed at what will happen and how easy and enjoyable it can be.

This doesn't mean for one second that once you change your brand all you will be able to eat is salad – so don't panic! Halfway through the book you could well start to think it's all about eating grass – that's why it's important to finish the whole book. Trust me, the amazing variety of beautiful foods you will be exposed to once you change your brand is in a different league to the bland, de-natured junkie-type foods you're on now.

I never dreamt that one day I would go out for a meal and actually *want* a main course fish or avocado salad – that I would choose it over everything else. I never thought that I would be in a position where I had the physical and mental energy to juice and blend every day – that it would become as automatic as having a shower in the morning. I never imagined that I would go out of my way and actually pass by McDonalds or Pizza Hut to get to a juice bar. I certainly never thought that I would look at people eating junk with genuine pity as opposed to total envy, as I used to on a diet. I just feel very lucky that I changed my brand of food when I did. I often wonder where I would be now if I hadn't.

CHANGING YOUR BRAND GIVES YOU CERTAINTY

I know for certain that I will never be overweight again. I know for certain I will never go on a diet. I know that I will not have to worry about whether I am getting the correct nutrients. I have energy, I feel light, I wake up and actually feel awake, I feel mentally sharp, I have regained confidence I had no idea I'd even lost, and I now wear whatever clothes I want. In short, I am what some people would describe as a 'health freak' and it is just simply the best feeling in the world.

The reason I have written this book is because I also know for certain that once you fully understand the food trap and follow a few simple instructions (my mental and physical 'recipe'), you too will change what you eat and you will love it. Everyone has it within their power to change their brand – because it's easy. Forget everything you have tried in the past and everything you have heard or read about food – let's start with a clean slate. No past to dwell on, just a compelling future to look forward to.

I have designed this book so that at the end you will not only want to change your brand, but you will literally love the process. And that tends to be the main problem people have when they think about changing what they eat. They feel all gloomy before they even start; as if they will be missing out and making a huge sacrifice by making the change. If you change your brand for life and totally change how you look at your old brand then you will never feel as though you are missing out for one simple reason – you will realize that you are not.

In order for you to see this clearly, and before we even attempt to make the change, we need to debunk the clap-trap that you've been bombarded with for years. 'Stuff' that is now stored in your head. We believe a lot of it because it is put across by 'experts'. But is it possible that some of the experts were taught incorrectly themselves? Is it possible that we just have too much information about food and nutrition? Is it possible that we have literally been blinded by science?

It's time to simplify this whole business about what we should eat, what quantity we should eat, what time we should eat and what is best for us by unloading our minds of pieces of so-called vital information, which plain and simply…

4

We Don't Need
to Know

What is your body fat ratio? What is your resting heart rate? Do you know? What is a bioflavonoid? What is riboflavin? Do you know? How many calories are there in a banana? How much protein do you need daily? How many vitamins are there? What is the best source of calcium? What does vitamin K do for you? Which has more vitamin C – an orange or a green pepper? What is a ketone? How does ketosis work? Do you know which foods contain vitamin P? What is your body mass index? What is your metabolic rate? If you do not know the answer to these questions – good! We don't need to know.

A little over one hundred years ago we didn't even know what a vitamin was, but we still got here didn't we? A gorilla doesn't know how many vitamins or minerals there are in a banana or whether it contains any calcium or protein: why don't they know? Because they don't need to know.

There are no nutritionists or dieticians in the wild. Oh, the poor creatures of this world, how do they cope? It almost makes you wonder how on earth they know what, and when, to eat. The fact is we do not wonder how they know. We expect them to know. So why do we not expect to know these simple things for ourselves? Why is there so much confusion over what we should eat, when is the best time to eat and at what point we should stop eating? The answer is simply too much knowledge, too much advertising, too much peer pressure, too many books and too much brainwashing from people with vested interests.

There is no advertising, brainwashing or 'intellectual' knowledge in the wild. Animals eat the 'brand of food' that was meant for them, they eat when they are genuinely hungry (the best time surely?) and they stop when they are full. They are perfectly happy eating their brand – it furnishes their body with everything they need and they love the taste and smell. Wild animals are also not concerned about how much they weigh, or what size fur they are. They don't worry, because they don't have to worry. All of their own kind are the same size and shape. If a giraffe became fat, tired and lethargic, would we need to test its blood pressure or put it on a scale to see if something was wrong with it? Or would we just know?

When I look back it seems strange that despite being a reasonably intelligent person, I would jump on a set of scales to see if I was overweight. Did I not already know? The only reason I jumped on them in the first place was because I already knew. But I just wanted to know by how much. Again, could I not see by how much? Did my bulges not tell me? All the scales do is confirm what you already know. I would even get on the scales slowly at times. Did I honestly think that by getting on the scales slowly I would not be as fat as I was? – that my scales would give a different reading? I believe all the 'intellectual' knowledge we are bombarded with makes us do things that are completely insane. Talking of which, here's a perfectly true story which illustrates what I mean. A friend of mine was on one of her many 'diets' some years back. On visiting her about a week or so into her 'new' diet, I noticed that there was a large chocolate cake, half eaten, on a plate next to her. To be honest I was quite glad because I know what a complete waste of time diets are. I asked her if she was still on her diet (assuming she wasn't) and to my surprise she said 'yes'. I said what about the half-eaten cake? What I heard next has gone down in history: 'It's okay', she explained 'because I weighed myself before I ate it and I weighed myself afterwards and guess what? – there was not an ounce of difference'. I wish I was joking, but that really is a true story.

I realize that most people haven't done something as mad as that, but there are hundreds, if not thousands, of perfectly intelligent people going somewhere on a weekly basis and actually paying for someone to weigh them – paying for someone to tell them what they already know. Although it may not seem like it at first glance, it is certainly on par with the half a cake thing.

I went to Weight Watchers many years ago for a couple of meetings. The 'leader' was actually very good and a very nice person. But what were we all doing there, weighing ourselves? At the time I attended if someone had lost weight from the week before, they would ring a bell and the group would do what I call a 'Ricky Lake'; they would literally clap and yell. Now I am all for encouraging and giving praise, but what about those who hadn't lost any weight. You feel bad enough as it is going in to one of those places – the last thing you need is to be made an object of pity. I am aware that Weight Watchers no longer do the bell thing, but they do still weigh you, along with nearly every other diet group.

Scales chain you to a diet mentality and they can be deceptive. Sometimes people look slimmer and feel healthier, but when they jump on the scales they see little or no change and so start to feel depressed. But sod the scales, it's how you look and feel that is the real measure of success. What many people fail to take into account is that…

Fat takes up five times more room on the body than muscle but muscle is a lot heavier than fat

So if you drop some fat but increase your muscle, your scales could well stay the same. So quit the scales and go for the 'look and feel' measure of success – it's a lot more accurate.

We not only use scales to weigh ourselves, but also to weigh the food we eat. And I don't mean for a recipe, I mean when we are on any kind of calorie counting diet. Why do we do this? Are we all a couple of grams short of an ounce?

A CALORIE IS A CALORIE IS A LOAD OF TOSH

The problem is that we have seen people doing these things for years so we just tend to follow suit without questioning what we are doing. Calories mean nothing. What is a calorie anyway? It's actually the amount of energy (heat) needed to raise one gram of water by one degree centigrade. In other words – we don't need to know. Again there is not one wild animal alive that knows how many calories are in the food they are eating for the same simple reason – they do not need to know. If you are thinking that we are better off knowing, ask yourself why? We apparently know more about 'nutrition' now than ever before, yet heart disease is still the number one killer disease in Western society.

We not only worry about this nutrition 'stuff' but industries have been built on our fears. We spend around £320m on vitamin and mineral tablets every year in the UK alone. And for what? To try and counter the effects of the processed and de-natured food we are consuming. But what about the pills themselves, haven't they also been processed? Aren't they also de-natured?

There are 40,000 phytochemicals in one tomato. What is a phyto-chemical? A name for a vitamin that they haven't formally named yet. Are there really 40,000 vitamins in one tomato? I don't actually know and I don't care because as long as I get it into my body, I don't need to know. Your body doesn't care whether you call them vitamins, minerals, bioflavonoids or zookinoids – it simply wants them and needs them.

Fruits and vegetables, as a whole, contain every single vitamin and mineral that we have found a name for and many more we haven't. They apparently keep finding new and amazing disease-fighting agents in all fruit and veg. Recently they've discovered some real beauties. Ever heard of beta-carotene? Well now they've found alpha-carotene. They have also discovered phenols, indoles, aromatic isothiocyanates, terpenes and organo-sulphur: all of which are part of the *new* category of 'anutrients'. NEW? They can shove together whatever letters they like but what they have found is not *new*. They seem to want to get the credit for something nature produces. Fruits, vegetables and nuts have been the same since the dawn of time and everything we need to furnish our bodies are to be found within them. When they do discover a 'new' phytochemical in a fruit or veg they tend to try to isolate it, extract it, recreate it, process it and put it in a pill. That is the equivalent of taking just one spark plug and the oil from a car in the belief you have found the most important components of a motor car because it can't run without them.

BLAH! BLAH! BLAH!

Most of the time 'they' also try and blind us with science by using what I call blah, blah, blah language. I am talking about people who will use the longest most obscure words available to describe something which is actually very simple. However, they have studied it for many years, have spent flipping great wedges of cash on their education and are going to let you know they have by completely losing you. Here is what scientist R.W. Stout wrote in 1985 to prove his point about something (I am yet to figure out what): 'The arterial wall is an insulin-sensitive tissue. Insulin promotes proliferation of arterial smooth muscle cells and enhances lipid synthesis and low density lipoprotein (LDL) receptor activity'. What the hell is he banging on about?

It is about time we all took our brainwashed heads out of the sand. We just do not need to know what our ideal weight is (according to some man-made scale). We should not be weighing our food to see how much to eat. Nor do we need to concern ourselves with vitamins, minerals, bioflavonoids, our body fat ratio, or our resting heart rate. It is time to simplify the whole business of eating and health, remove the fear of changing, and find physical and mental freedom for life. We will not achieve this by worrying about vitamin K, B_6, C, D, K, Z, protein, calcium, or what foods are low fat. We will achieve our goal for life by *not* concerning ourselves with all this nonsense, but by removing the many years of brainwashing and relying on ourselves.

You already know why you shouldn't be eating the foods you are and why you should eat the foods you are not. However, that doesn't matter because everybody with a food problem consciously knows this, yet this knowledge does not help them. It certainly didn't help me. All it did was add pressure and make me feel stupid and weak-willed. What would I do if I was under pressure or feeling down? EAT!

The problem is that although we know all the benefits of making the change, we also believe that we have to go through *pain* to get there and stay there. As I will repeat throughout this book, you will not have to endure any pain at all because it's easy to lose weight, gain health, have the body of your dreams and all the energy to enjoy it. You simply need to get into the right frame of *mind*, then you can easily get into the right frame of *body*. You will only have to suffer a lifetime of pain if you don't make the change – not if you do.

By now you should realize what you don't need to know, but in order to remove all the brainwashing and release you from certain 'drug foods', there is a lot you do need to know. The first and most important thing is the nature of the food trap. What really compels us to eat things that we then regret eating almost instantaneously? What makes us eat foods that we know for certain are *causing* excess fat, ill health, depression, stress and premature death? In other words…

5

Why *do* People Eat Junk Food?

 The answer is very simple. It is a combination of just two reasons:

1 The advertising, brainwashing and conditioning we have been subjected to since birth (the mental side).
2 An empty insecure physical feeling due to malnutrition, low blood sugar, or a combination of the two – caused by the 'food' itself (the physical side).

These two factors add up to addiction.

The good news is that any kind of addiction is easy to kick once you understand how that particular addiction works – which is what this book is all about. The addiction to any kind of food is mainly psychological: the physical effect, which often triggers the mental cravings, is very easy to overcome. In fact, with the help of what I call 'the fastest food in the west' bringing sunshine to every cell in the body, you will hardly notice any physical symptoms of withdrawal.

The main problem is the first of the two factors: the many, many years of conditioning, brainwashing and total misinformation that we have been subjected to by the advertisers and so-called experts. This is really the *cause* of the problem and this is what needs to be fully removed. The lethargy, weight gain, health problems etc. are simply *symptoms* of the cause. You must learn to think before you put food into your mouth. It is time to wake up and realize that the livelihoods of many people depend on keeping us none the wiser when it comes to just how harmful and addictive certain foods can be. It is often their job to keep you hooked – without your knowledge of course – on what I will continue to refer to as drug foods. They are constantly trying to change the way you think in order to give you the very false impression that *you* are choosing to eat and drink their drug foods.

The tobacco companies played the same game for years. They kept very quite about the fact that their product is addictive, controls lives and kills people – and all the while it was advertised on television and radio (and of course the government got its share of the profits). Cigarette ads may have disappeared from the small screen but product placement for smoking in the film industry is still very prevalent.

Is it possible the same thing is happening with the so-called 'food' industry? There is even a McDonalds in the grounds of the Tower of London. As if that wasn't outrageous enough, McDonalds even have one of their 28,000 outlets in Guy's hospital in London. Yes, a hospital! McDonalds have a policy which states that they want everybody to be within 4 minutes of one of their – and I use the term loosely – restaurants at any time.

'But Jasey, you cannot put junk food in the same category as cigarettes. Cigarettes kill people, control their lives, cost them a fortune and are addictive.'

So where exactly is the difference? As a nation the UK spends £25bn a year on fast food – that's £7m a day. Second only to the US. This money is spent on 'foods' that are *known* to be addictive and are *known* to cause all kinds of diseases, including heart disease – the number one killer in Western society. Table salt is known to kill over 40,000 people a year in the UK, that's over 100 people a day. This is virtually the same number as alcohol, yet there is no warning on the label at all. Come to think of it there is no warning on alcohol either. White refined carbohydrates and refined sugar are *known* to be a major cause of diabetes and a whole host of other diseases (which I will explain later). Aspartame (the artificial sweetener found in diet drinks etc.) has been linked to all kinds of health problems. It is known to tighten blood vessels, cause additional thirst and has been linked to brain tumours. Yet not only is it being sold as a 'food' stuff, but is promoted as a product that will *help* people if they have a weight problem. (I will cover aspartame and products like it in depth later so you'll never want to touch them again.)

The point is this, in my estimation 'drug foods' and 'junk food' overall actually kill more people than all other drugs combined. And yes that includes heroin, crack, cocaine and even cigarettes. Yet there is not one single drug food or junk food product that has a warning on it.

We get uptight because cigarette companies are still allowed to spend £120m a year in the UK advertising a product that is known to kill more than one in three of its customers. Yet the fast food and junk food industries spend literally billions advertising products that are *known* to be a major cause of diabetes, obesity, heart disease and liver failure – to name but a few. These are 'foods' that can and *do* cause premature death, just like cigarettes; control people's lives, just like cigarettes; and products which, I estimate, slowly kill 2 in 3 of those who are hooked on them (which is *more* than cigarettes).

You cannot open a magazine, switch on your TV, or go to the cinema without being bombarded with images of drug-type foods. The government of course is not about to do anything about it as they earn billions in tax revenue from people's addictions to these heart-disease causing, stroke-inducing so-called foods. Their argument is always the same and runs along the lines of people are not stupid, they know the facts, we advise them to eat five portions of fruit and veg a day – if they choose to eat junk, then it's up to them. Yet they make it law to wear a seat belt. Why isn't it our choice then? Because people are not addicted to putting on or leaving off their seat belts, but they are addicted to trashy foods. To say to someone like Barry Austin, who I believe, at the age of 29, was 50st in weight and had a 82in waist[1], that it's his genuine choice to be like that is ludicrous. Given the genuine

[1] *Daily Mail* article 8/10/97

choice I imagine he would love to end his addiction to trash foods; he would love to be slim.

One of the major problems with 'food' addiction is that the problem is *visible* because the main symptom is excess fat. Think about it: no matter how many cigarettes someone smokes, they're never called a black tar, nicotine-filled git or a cigarette-smoking bastard are they? Yet along with food addiction go the names and the scathing attack on our characters: we get called gits and pigs – we're never just fat. This is why so many people don't reach obesity – because of how they will look. But they still have a food problem and are still constantly battling to control what they eat.

I used to feel very proud of myself if I managed to be good for a few days, or if I managed to control my intake of chocolate to the point where I only had it at weekends. I often used to cut down on the coffee and biscuits – put myself on the 'food wagon' if you will. There are people who do manage to exercise control over their intake of trash food, but this is an awful way to go through life. If you have to exercise control over something, it must mean that that something is controlling you. It is the need to exercise control that means you are *not* in control. Confused? Let me put it this way. I do not have to exercise control over my banana intake, if I needed to discipline myself with my bananas then I would have a banana problem. For years smokers thought it was their genuine choice to smoke (in fact some people still retain this belief). However, when the smoker was forced to stand outside their workplace in the freezing cold in order to get their fix, they started to realize they were not *choosing* to smoke, but *had* to (I know first-hand as I used to smoke 40–50 a day).

I do not know one single person who has to exercise control over their sardine intake. Why? Because it is not a drug-like food. I also don't know anyone who would have the slightest problem getting rid of sardines from their diet if a doctor told them they caused heart disease, lethargy, weight gain and premature death. Yet there are hundreds of thousands of people who, if you told them the same thing about coffee, chocolate, or fast-food burgers for example, would say, 'Up yours, life's too short' and continue eating them. Why? Because they are drug-like foods that compel people to want more and more. Whether they actually have more and more is neither here nor there, it's *wanting* more that causes the real problem – the need to exercise control.

TOTALLY WIRED

Some unfortunate people have lost the ability to exercise control over what they eat or drink. It was reported[2] that Barry Austin was told he would die unless he slimmed, and he went through the drastic measure of having his stomach stapled. I also understand that when he was 19 he had his jaws wired together which lasted for four months and he lost four stone in that time because all he could consume was soup. I imagine his life was hell, especially at Christmas when he saw all the beautiful food laid out in front of him and knew he couldn't take part. Can you imagine the torture he must have been going through? Apparently, his family liquidized his roast dinner and pudding for him to drink but on seeing the mush he was supposed to drink, his desperation was such that he ripped the wires out with wire cutters, leaving his mouth bleeding in agony. Do you think he goes through all this for a hamburger because he simply likes the taste? Is it possible that there is more to it? Is it possible he is simply mentally and physically addicted to drug foods in the same way a nicotine addict is addicted to cigarettes? It is not just possible but obvious. It is not his genuine choice to do this – given the choice he would just eat healthily. Is it also possible that something is controlling his thought process?

The reason I have used Barry (who had been, reportedly, the fattest man in Britain) as an example is to illustrate the point that often it is not our genuine choice to eat certain 'foods'. We have simply been conditioned or brainwashed to the point where we get upset and even angry if we feel we can no longer do it. Unless you start to realize what is going on, you are in danger of remaining in the food trap for life. The point of this book is to set you mentally free, so that you can eat whatever you want to and not what someone has conditioned you to in order to boost their bank balance. This can only happen if you fully understand how the people peddling drug and junk foods go about their business.

[2] *Daily Mail* article 8/10/97

AD – FABRICATED

How do you sell a product that is of very dubious quality, is unhealthy and is contributing to (and in many cases causing) major health problems. Good old advertising of course. We have literally been programmed and conditioned to consume trash foods and drinks. That is why people think it's normal to eat these foods. But then didn't people think it was normal and sociable to smoke a few years ago too?

Let us not underestimate the power of all the advertising and conditioning either: it works. Our brains are very clever computers, but they can be literally programmed just like any other computer. Unless we learn to run it effectively ourselves, there are many, many people who are paid tremendous amounts of money to run it for us – and they do. That is why we have such a strong belief that fruit and veg are for boring people who don't want to 'live'. After all with Pepsi Max you can go snowboarding, skiing, bungee jumping and 'Live life to the max – Pepsi Max'. Then of course we all know that 'A Mars A Day helps you work rest and play' and that 'Breakfast at McDonalds makes your day'. I can't ever remember hearing 'Live life to the max with a fresh mouthwatering Mango Max' or 'An apple a day helps you work, rest, play and helps prevent cancer' or 'Breakfast at a juice bar, stimulates the mind, feeds the cells, helps to lift the waste from your body and really does make your day that little more alive and vibrant'. Incidentally, if breakfast at McDonalds does make your day – YOU REALLY DO NEED THIS BOOK.

THE BELLS

Ivan Pavlov's famous experiment illustrated just how easily we can be conditioned. It has been well documented, but for those of you who are not aware of the experiment I will explain it briefly. He starved his pet dog for three days, then, when he gave it some food, he rang a bell at the same time. After that, every time his dog felt genuine hunger, Ivan would put some food down and at exactly the same time he would ring a bell. He didn't simply do this once or twice, but over and over again until it became a conditioned response: food/bell, food/bell, food/bell. In the end (and this is why I am using this analogy) even if the dog had *already* eaten and could have in no way felt genuine physical hunger, when the bell was rung the dog would look for food and literally begin to salivate.

Advertisers for drug and junk food know the power of this and they use it to sell you food when you are not even hungry. Have you ever been driving along, not even thinking about food, when all of a sudden you saw the two golden arches of the McDonalds sign and felt hungry? Or do you remember when you were a kid playing in the street, not thinking of food at all, when all of a sudden you heard the sound of the ice cream man and decided you felt hungry? WELL THAT'S THE BELL. Going to the cinema means popcorn and a drink: THAT'S THE BELL. Easter – a chocolate egg: THAT'S THE BELL. Christmas – turkey or pudding: THAT'S THE BELL. It's 11.30am – time for a Diet Coke break : THAT'S THE BELL. Going to get petrol? – time for a pastie, or a bar of chocolate and soft drink: THAT'S THE BELL. Elevenses – time for a cup of tea (and a biscuit of course): THAT'S THE BELL.

The fact is we react to a thousand different bells without realizing it. The way they link in a bell is to advertise it over and over again. Sometimes they even include a specific time to take their product (as in the case of Diet Coke – 11.30am). This is why they pay people like Robbie Williams, Madonna and the Spice Girls millions for a 30 second commercial to advertise products like Pepsi-cola. They link their 'feel good' music to a product that has nothing to do with feeling good.

I was giving a seminar recently where I asked a young lady why she drank Diet Coke. She said, and I quote word for word, 'I drink it just for the taste of it'. Can you remember what the slogan for Diet Coke was or still is? It was sung like this 'just for the taste of it – Diet Coke'. This was the slogan and this young woman has been 'belled' so much that she now believes it is her genuine opinion. She did not hear 'just for the taste of it' once, but over and over and over again until it was linked in her brain. That is the only way to create a bell. They must beam their message over and over again. If they didn't we would forget their message.

Do you remember this?

'When your carpet smells fresh your room does too so every time you vacuum remember what to do. Do the shake and vac and put the freshness back, do the shake and vac and put the freshness back'.

I would be surprised if you don't, because it was the most successful advertising campaign of all time for a household cleaner. The point I am making is that you haven't heard or seen this particular advert for at least 21 years yet you remember it like it was yesterday – why? Because they beamed the song again and again and again until in the end you couldn't help but sing it and buy the product. This is why I make no apologies for repeating certain points throughout this book. It is the only way to remove the bells and create new empowering ones. So if you think, 'He's said that already' – I know, it was intentional!

The products we are dealing with here are not household cleaners, but ones that can literally destroy people's quality of life and reduce their life expectancy. They are products which – if consumed in large enough quantities – have been proven to undermine confidence, depress and disable people. They can also enslave them. Oh, and of course, let's not forget that in the long run they can also kill you.

We are constantly being bombarded with so many 'trendy' images of junk food. The junk food outlets have all become fashion statements. We have McDonalds, Burger King, Pizza Hut, KFC, Ben and Jerry's, Häagen-Dazs, Starbucks, and Cadburys, to name just a few. It has literally become a 'designer label' business. Is it any wonder that so many people are under the misapprehension that junk is where the pleasure is? that trash foods are a treat and fruit and veg are boring? Things have got so bad that we now believe that it is 'normal' to eat this rubbish and 'abnormal' to eat healthily.

These images and beliefs have been drip-fed into our computer brains since we were born. Of all the bells, these are the most detrimental. Many television programmes and virtually all Hollywood films are also playing their part. Product placement is huge in the film and television industry, especially for drug-like foods and drinks. The coffee chain Starbucks, for instance, are now a major placement in many of the Hollywood Blockbusters. The movie *You Got Mail* should have been called *You Got Starbucks*. Hollywood has an entire department devoted to product placement, and specific agents to get your product in the latest blockbuster. And if they can get the actor to drink or eat the product it's a hit. It's one thing getting Superman thrown into a huge Coke sign, but if they can get him to drink it – BINGO! In the film Austin Powers, the lead actor mentioned Heineken and sales of the beer went up by 15 per cent – hardly a coincidence.

They all sell the idea that you can feed emotion and make yourself happy with their product. If someone's boyfriend leaves them on a TV show, the first thing to come out is the ice cream. If a child is depressed we can cheer them up with a chocolate bar or 'treat' them to a McDonalds. The problem is that we end up believing it. Not only that, but we *all* play our part in keeping the chain going: 'Tidy your room and you can have an ice cream', 'If you are good, you can have a chocolate bar', or perhaps worst of all 'If you eat your vegetables, you can have a treat'.

We have all been conditioned to believe that junk is a reward, a treat, a comforter and a genuine pleasure from a very early age; and sadly those who care for us most are often the biggest culprits. To compound the message we have sounds and images beamed into our computer brains confirming what we have been taught. Every holiday seems to have a strong bell that revolves around food: Easter means chocolate eggs, birthdays mean cakes, Christmas equals pudding and so on.

The main reason why most people in Western society are caught in the food trap is because it is an exceptionally easy one for people to fall into. Years ago it was very easy for people to fall into the smoking trap. This was largely down to everyone believing it was not only okay to smoke at the time, but that it was very sociable and had no harmful effects (well the masses believed that – the people in the know always knew). Everyone now knows that smoking causes cancer, and it is widely seen as anti-social. The nicotine companies therefore have to work harder and harder to get people hooked on their product.

However, unlike 'real' drugs, drug foods are seen as *genuine* food, and most of us have been on this junkie stuff from a very early age. In fact, if you were not breast fed there is a good chance you have been on junkie and drug foods ever since you were born. Even if you weren't on rubbish from the second you left the womb, it wouldn't have been long before you had your first fix.

Think about it – at what age would you give a child a cigarette? Never I guess, but 16 at the earliest. What about an alcoholic drink? Well it varies, but usually we wouldn't dream of anything less than double figures. What about junkie or drug food? Ah, now we begin to see the problem. It seems perfectly *normal* to feed children junk and drug foods from a very early age. Not only is it seen as normal, but this drug-like food is seen as a treat; as a reward – so much so that you are seen as a baddie if you refuse to give them some. At the same time we are bombarded with billions of pounds worth of advertising that is cleverly designed to keep people hooked on (or to change their brand of) drug-like food.

The biggest problem, and this is where you really need to open your mind, is that the so-called food itself seems to confirm everything we believe. Our minds are often easily deluded because of a physical chemical reaction in our body – a reaction which seems to confirm the advertiser's message and what we believe to be true. As I have mentioned previously, there are two sides to the food trap: mental and physical. Over 95 per cent of the 'food' problem is in reality mental. However, in order for us to see through the illusions of the food trap we need to forget the mental for a second and…

6

Let's Get Physical

As you are no doubt aware, all businesses are out to increase their profits. How does any business sell more of the same product to the same person? Simple: by making them believe that they need it, that it will benefit them, and that their life would be incomplete in some way without it. The drug food industry is no different. They will do anything and say anything to get you literally hooked on their brand of drug food.

'But how can they do this with food?' you ask. 'You're either hungry or you're not. And if you're hungry, you eat and you're then satisfied, body and mind – end of story'. Yes, that is the nature of *real, natural* food, as I now realize. But, as we've all experienced, that is not how we feel after eating rubbish. These foods often do the complete opposite: we feel anything but satisfied after eating them, and this is why people are hooked. It's very similar to how cigarette addiction works. The tobacco companies would have made very little money if a smoker had just one cigarette a day. How do they make them have more? Well they don't really have to do a great deal; the drug will do most of it for them.

JUST AN ILLUSION

When nicotine leaves the body it creates an empty insecure feeling, rather like a hunger for food. The feeling is so slight the smoker does not realize that the previous cigarette they had caused the feeling. They have another one and the empty insecure feeling goes away. They no longer feel as low, as empty or as insecure as they did, and so end up believing there is a genuine pleasure in smoking. Yet all they are enjoying is the ending of an aggravation which was caused by the previous cigarette. All the tobacco industry then had to do was some product placement and advertising. Words such as 'smooth' and 'satisfaction' were used to describe cigarette smoking on advertisements. Every film and television hero was a smoker etc. As most people are aware, the body will always build up an immunity and tolerance to any drug and you therefore end up needing more and more to get the same effect. In the end a feeling of dissatisfaction is felt even when the addict is taking the drug. The nicotine companies found a way to create an *additional* hunger to a normal hunger and certain members of the 'food' industry have done exactly the same thing with some foods – drug foods to be specific. Now just in case this is starting to sound a tad blah, blah, blahish, I want to explain in simple terms the difference between a drug food, a junk food and a natural food.

Drug food

Any 'food' that contains 'empty' nutrients, has virtually no enzyme activity, does not feed the body, and which creates either feelings of withdrawal, or high then low blood sugar (what most people would describe as junk food such as sugar).

A group of foods which create a *false* need, a *false* hunger – a compulsion to have more of the same.

Junk food

Any food that contains some or no nutrients, but does *not* create feelings of withdrawal or low blood sugar (what some people think of as natural food such as meat, cheese, fish, etc.).

A group of foods which do not create a false need, but can be hard work for the body to use, digest and dispose of.

Natural food

Any food that contains *live* nutrients, genuinely feeds the body, and takes little or no work for the body to digest, assimilate and dispose of.

A group of foods which are in their natural state – as nature intended.

Drug foods are the real cause of the food trap. They are designed to create *additional* hungers and feelings of *dissatisfaction* – the complete opposite of natural foods. I must point out that both drug and junk foods slowly starve the human body, especially when they are at the cost of natural foods. The sad reality is that most people are suffering from malnutrition. In fact whenever you see someone who is overweight you can be almost certain they are suffering from this condition. When we think of malnutrition, we tend to see images of starving people in the developing world, so it's hard to imagine that someone who eats loads of food is also suffering from it. But the fact is they are.

WHAT IS MALNUTRITION?

The Oxford dictionary describes it as 'A dietary condition resulting from the absence of some foods or the absence of essential elements necessary for health; insufficient nutrition'. This is exactly what I was suffering from when I was over 30lb overweight, and it is what every junk and drug food addict is suffering from whether they are overweight or not. They have a severe lack of nutrients going into the body. Without nutrients feeding the cells, the body will of course be hungry. No wonder junk and drug food addicts feel hungry and dissatisfied a lot of the time: it's because they are. If the body doesn't get what it needs it *stays* hungry for nutrients. Hunger is not a pleasant feeling, it's an empty, insecure, dissatisfied feeling. What do you do when you feel hungry, empty and dissatisfied? EAT!

It is this simple:

The less food you eat containing live nutrients, the *hungrier* you will become. The hungrier you become the more *dissatisfied* and *incomplete* you will feel. The more dissatisfied and incomplete you feel the *more* you eat to try and feel satisfied and complete.

This, in itself, is bad enough. However, an even greater problem we have are the *additional* hungers we experience on top of genuine hunger. These are caused by drug foods; and the empty, insecure feelings they produce feel identical to a normal, genuine hunger. Such feelings are the result of the withdrawal effects from certain drug foods, or the effects of low blood sugar – which, again, are caused by the drug foods themselves. You will not get these false hungers from what I define as junk foods (I will give plenty of examples of junk food later, so by the time you finish this book the three main Juice Master food groups will be crystal clear).

Drug foods really are a double whammy. Not only do they contain *nothing* of any use to the body whatsoever, they ultimately create a set of false hungers which feel exactly the same as a normal genuine hunger. And because they are sold as food, and not drugs, people remain none the wiser to the fact they are hooked on a drug. Instead, people who are caught in the food trap because of drug foods are called 'pigs', and are often ostracized and given no sympathy whatsoever.

It is the *false* physical hungers, along with the advertising, which cause people to have mental cravings for drug foods.

This is ultimately why people attempt to 'use' drug foods in much the same way drug addicts attempt to 'use' drugs: i.e. reaching for them in times of boredom, loneliness, or for comfort etc. That is what causes the food trap. What frustrates me most is that the people who make and distribute drug foods even have the front to advertise the fact that their product will *not* end a genuine hunger. They have the audacity to let us know that their 'food' will only seemingly satisfy a *false* mental and physical hunger. Our problem is that we don't question it because we believe it's our choice and that we derive some genuine pleasure from it. A great example of this was an advert for a chocolate bar which claimed you could 'Eat it in-between meals without ruining your appetite'. So what's the point of eating it then?

I thought the whole point of eating was to *satisfy* your appetite, to *end* your hunger. With this advert they are blatantly telling us that their 'food' will not satisfy a genuine hunger. In other words it won't feed you. Another old ad that did this was the finger of fudge one. If you cannot recall allow me, 'It's full of Cadbury goodness and very small to eat, a finger of fudge is just enough until it's time to eat.' First of all what the hell do they mean by goodness. It makes me wonder how they still manage to get away with such rubbish. The second part says, 'it's just enough until it's time to eat.' In other words it's just enough to take the edge off the *false* hunger, but it won't ruin your *genuine* appetite.

The reason we are so easily fooled is not because we are stupid, but because such products do feed the *false* hungers; in the same way nicotine feeds a smoker's hunger for nicotine and heroin feeds a heroin addict's hunger for heroin. When you end any kind of hunger you feel a sense of relief. A feeling of relief from any type of aggravation is pleasurable and this is where the confidence trick really kicks in. The makers and advertisers of these so-called foods try to give the impression that there is a *genuine* pleasure in eating, even if you are not genuinely hungry. But it is a *false* sense of pleasure created by a *false* hunger. On top of that you've got every diet and 'health' book giving the advice over and over again that you should simply 'eat when you feel hungry'. But the point I am making is that the drug food eater has additional hungers and is hungry, but it is a false hunger created by the rubbish itself – they are effectively in a loop.

Until the drug food addict realizes exactly what's going on, statements like 'eat only when you feel hungry' are ludicrous. Someone like Tierney Woods – who, at the age of 15, weighed in at 41st 12lb – was no doubt following the advice to eat only when hungry, but she was such a drug food addict and had built up an immunity to drug foods to such a degree that she probably felt the false hungers even when she was stuffing herself with drug foods in her desperation to relieve her false hungers. At this stage she would be in a constant state of withdrawal, would be hypoglycaemic and have a constant level of insulin in her blood (which, as I will explain in simple terms later, can cause a permanent state of dissatisfaction). And this condition was seemingly only lessened to some degree by more drug foods.

And once again the makers and advertisers of drug foods play on this feature of their product –

'Nothing seems to satisfy like a Snickers'

This was another advertising slogan blatantly informing the drug food addict that nothing will satisfy their need like a drug food. Why? Because their need is a false one created by the drug food in the first place. Let me explain. All the food in the world will never satisfy a smoker's physical and psychological need for nicotine. All the *food* in the world will never satisfy a heroin addict's physical and psychological need for heroin. Why? Because they are completely *separate* hungers created by the drug itself. Non-smokers and non-heroin addicts just do not have these hungers. This point is obvious when we are talking about what people clearly regard as drugs, but it is exactly the same with drug foods. And this is why it is essential to really open your mind and change the way you view these 'foods' – it is a vital part of solving your food problem for life.

All the *natural* food in the world will never satisfy a physical and/or psychological need for drug food. Why? Because it is a false physical and mental hunger that has fooled us all for generations. That is why you can seemingly satisfy your *false* need for junk without ruining your *genuine* appetite. It explains why even when I did eat fruit or salad it just didn't seem to satisfy me the same way as junk and drug food. And it also explains why I would sometimes feel stuffed but, at the same time, dissatisfied and still hungry. This is one of the most important points in this book and it will be repeated at certain times to hammer home the message. I make no apologies for some of the repetition in this book. I want you to have excellent health, physical and mental vibrancy, the body of your dreams and, more importantly, freedom to eat what you want, when you want – *not* what someone else has conditioned you to eat. I also want you to get more *genuine* pleasure from eating and drinking than you have had in your entire life. This can only happen for life if you get the message and see behind the nonsense we have been bombarded with over the years.

The excellent news is that the false hungers are very easy to get rid of and towards the end of the book I will discuss how to starve them to death and enjoy the process. First you need a full understanding of drug foods and false hungers. There are several products that create false hungers and I will cover each in turn. However, the biggest culprit of false hunger, the biggest drug food of them all and what really compels people to overeat and to eat as a response to emotion is a substance which, when it hits your bloodstream, has your body screaming…

7

Oh Sugar!

 'Sugar…, ah honey, honey, you are my candy girl, and you got me wanting you'

No, I haven't gone barking mad, it just seems that whoever wrote that song was a sugar addict. I'm just kidding of course, but the words 'you got me wanting you' is very accurate for the average sugar addict.

Sugar not only needs a chapter to itself, but an entire book could be written on this subject. We do not have time for that and you really do not need to know the entire history of the sugar industry to rid it from your life. All you need to know is what really happens when you eat white refined sugar.

When natural food is eaten, it is first broken down in the mouth then passed into the stomach. Once there it is further broken down and eventually passed into the intestines, where the energy and nutrients can slowly be absorbed. The body then has the job of getting rid of the waste through the usual outlets – bowels, bladder, lungs, skin, etc. White refined sugar is very different. It goes straight through the stomach wall *without* being digested, giving an instant rush of glucose to the bloodstream. This causes your blood sugar levels to rise too high. You now have too much sugar in your blood and (what they call) your 'PH balance' is out of sorts (this is not to be confused with your skin PH). Your blood PH level is very, very important. If it goes just a couple of points below or above what it should be you will die. Your body therefore has to do whatever it can to counteract your rocketing blood sugar levels and reinstate the body's normal balance. How does it do this? By robbing some of your body's bank account of the powerful hormone insulin. Any rush that you feel when you have sugar is simply the rush of insulin entering the bloodstream to try and counteract the excess sugar you have just put in. The insulin produced to deal with this high blood sugar causes your blood sugar levels to fall. And when you feel the effects of low blood sugar what do you need? A quick fix. The moment the insulin reaction has cleansed your bloodstream of this excess sugar, you will be running on empty – an empty feeling created by sugar. This white refined trash has no nutrients, vitamins, minerals, essential fats or amino acids. In other words it contains not one single ingredient that genuinely feeds the human body. It contains NOTHING, not a sausage, not even a chipolata. It is a totally empty so-called food that leaves *you* feeling empty. It is, however, used at every available opportunity by the drug food industry.

SUGAR CAUSES LOW BLOOD SUGAR

Remember – if your sugar levels were balanced you would feel satisfied for longer and the hunger you feel would always be a genuine one. Now, that's simply no good for the refined sugar industry – they need you to feel the effects of low blood sugar, they want your sugar levels to crash, they want you to feel unbalanced. That way you will feel the need for a quick fix and thus the sugar industry is guaranteed repeat business. This is because the only thing that appears to end the feeling is white refined sugar – the very thing that *caused* the problem in the first place. It's like treating the symptoms of a disease with the cause. White refined sugar causes dis-ease in the body, which in turn causes dis-ease in the mind.

Many people I see are under the misapprehension that they don't consume that much sugar. If they don't have it in their tea, coffee, or on their cereal, they assume there is little sugar in their diet. However, this substance is in virtually every processed food we consume. It's a great filler and it also prolongs shelf life (perhaps the only life that is ever prolonged because of sugar). Plus it tastes sweet so they can easily fool us into believing we are continuing to eat this rubbish simply because we love the taste and that it is our choice.

I must make this next point very clear – when I talk about sugar, I am not just talking about the stuff found in 'soft' drinks, processed foods, chocolate, cakes, ketchup, etc. I am also talking about white refined carbohydrates such as *white* rice, pasta, bread, cereals etc. which rapidly turn to glucose (sugar) in the bloodstream. We consume a vast amount of these and they are *all* empty, non-foods which send your blood sugar levels sky-high, causing the pancreas to produce more insulin. The fast food outlets – the ones who rake in £2.7bn a year in the UK from drug foods – use white refined trash in all forms to keep you coming back for more. They rely on the stuff. Without white refined sugars and salt (more on this topic later) they would go out of business – they would literally have nothing to sell apart from the round squashed piece of 'mystery' food which you find slammed in-between a white refined bun. (Incidentally, even a cockroach will only eat white bread in extreme emergencies.)

If you are overweight, unhealthy or both, then this chapter is one of the most important you will ever read in your life because the chances are…

White refined sugars and carbs are the drug-like foods that are a major cause of your problem

When you eat white refined bread, pasta, rice, flour etc. your sugar levels go up rapidly and more insulin is secreted to help counteract it. Any 'lift' you feel from a sugar or carbo 'hit' is very short lived and in no time you feel a drop as the body scrambles to balance its blood sugar levels. Something else too: the insulin that has been produced by the pancreas to rectify your blood sugar is also known as the 'fat-producing hormone'. Its job is to transport the carbohydrate energy (which has been converted by the body into glucose) to the liver and muscle cells for short-term storage of energy. However, if there is too much glucose at once – which is inevitable when white refined foods are consumed – some of the excess glucose has to go into the long-term storage banks: in other words it is stored as FAT.

Let me simplify to make this insulin, low blood sugar thing very clear. Insulin is produced by the pancreas to counteract the excess glucose (or sugar) that floods the bloodstream when you eat white refined foods. Any over-spill from the high amounts of insulin necessary to tackle this onslaught are stored as fat. When the insulin levels start to come down, a signal is sent to the brain that the sugar levels have now stabilized. Once the sugar levels stabilize, you feel satisfied. However, in no time at all, the blood sugar level *falls* as the food it was given was an empty fuel and one that is released into the blood much too quickly. So when your sugar levels drop again to an uncomfortable level, you once again get an empty dissatisfied feeling. If you then try and *satisfy* this feeling with more white refined trash, the cycle will continue. This loop is problematic enough and, along with the advertising, is what keeps people hooked. However, just like a drug addict who needs more and more of their drug to try and feel satisfied as time goes on, so it is for the white refined carbo/sugar addict.

Here's why:

If the carbo/sugar addict attempts to satisfy his or her hunger by eating more *white refined* carbs (simple or complex), the insulin amounts released by the pancreas will be even *greater* and the feeling of satisfaction becomes even less. As stated, it is only when the insulin levels *drop* that the person feels satisfied. So when you constantly consume these white refined 'foods' you end up always having a degree of insulin in your blood. This means *never* feeling truly satisfied and always feeling a slight void in your life. You become what is known as 'insulin resistant', meaning your body will need more insulin to maintain a normal blood sugar range than that of a person who is not insulin resistant. At the same time this process progressively lowers the level of serotonin in the brain. Apparently, serotonin is a neurotransmitter and this neurowhatsit helps to govern your mood. Too little and depression sets in. This means a white refined carbohydrate works just like any other drug. It makes you feel low, both mentally and physically, but gives the impression that it picks you up – clever trick, eh!

If you are reading this book in order to get a slim physique, then you need to realize that it's sugar, rather than fat, that is causing your problem. This may be a bold statement, but it's true. Here's why: after you eat refined sugar/carbs the insulin levels in your blood will usually stay quite high for several hours (remember, insulin is the fat-*producing* hormone). If you start your day with refined sugar/carbs (cereal, bagel, etc.), have them again in some form at lunch (sandwich and crisps), then again at night and maybe in a cup of something before you go to bed, the insulin levels in your blood can stay high for up to 16–18 hours a day! So what? Well picture this powerful hormone literally shoving fat into your cells 16–18 hours a day – not much time left in the day to for the body to break it down and shift it now is there?

The fact is we *do* need sugar and carbs; the human body was designed to get its energy from carbohydrates – but carbs that are in their natural state, not ones that have been stripped of their life force (or refined as they call it). I am talking here about natural fruits, vegetables and whole grains. Our bodies were never designed to deal with a constant barrage of white, refined rubbish. The body will, of course, 'survive' for quite a while despite this abuse – but it's the *quality* of our daily lives that is being slowly destroyed and controlled by these products. When you eat natural, nothing-taken-out carbs, the body does what it was designed to do. It digests them and then it *gradually* releases their potential energy into your cells. This does not cause your sugar levels to go sky high and therefore the pancreas does not have to produce tons of insulin. The sugar found in fruit is *fructose*. The body cannot use fructose as it is, and needs to convert it into usable glucose. The time it takes to convert the fructose into glucose is essential in keeping the blood sugar levels correctly balanced. Plus, fruit sugar is a whole food. It contains all the enzymes (life force) the body needs for digestion, it is a pure 'live' food, it tastes wonderful and also contains fibre, which helps to 'sweep' the intestines clean and helps to prevent the sugar being absorbed too rapidly into the bloodstream. White refined carbs do the complete opposite.

WHITE REFINED SUGAR – THE COCAINE OF THE FOOD WORLD

It's about time people started to realize that white refined sugar is not just like a drug, but is a drug – a drug which, just like any other, compels people to take more and more. However, unlike the other perfectly legal drugs like cigarettes, white refined sugar/carbs don't carry a government health warning – despite the fact that they are *known* by the medical profession to cause a multitude of diseases and have been heavily, and I do mean very heavily, linked to diabetes, hypertension in children and antisocial behaviour. Diabetes has more than tripled since 1958; right in line with the consumption of sugar – coincidence? A little over 100 years ago only one per cent of the population had diabetes, now the figure is officially 1 in 12; unofficially it's a lot more. There are many people who are unaware that they have what is known as type 2 diabetes (over 90 per cent of diabetics have this type: type 1 is where you inject yourself). As we now consume over a third of a pound of sugar each per day, the number of people suffering from this life-threatening condition can only rise. At present over 100 million people around the world have diabetes and that figure is projected to rise to a whopping 250 million by 2015. White refined sugar is also said to be responsible for the premature deaths of 3000 British women every year due to heart disease: 'Oh it's only a bit of sugar, you've got to live you know' – EXACTLY.

This same refined sugar is also the substance found in so many low fat foods – which seems ironic given that white refined sugar *causes* insulin release and insulin is the fat-*producing* hormone. Yet over the past twenty to thirty years people have come to believe that their weight and/or health problem will be solved for life if they simply went…

8

Fat Free

I know that not everyone reading this book is doing so in
order to lose weight, but there are so many people, fat or
otherwise, who continue to buy 'fat free' and 'low fat'
products in a bid for better health. I was guilty of this myself for years.
However, what they, and I, failed to realize is the simple truth –

It's all bullshit

Not only do these products nearly always contain more fat than is
stated on the label but, nine times out of ten, they are full of white
refined sugar. This kind of defeats the object of the exercise somewhat
don't you think? Do you know you could get a suitcase full of white
refined sugar and put a massive label on it reading '100% fat free'. And
the thing is you wouldn't be lying – it is totally fat free. The fact that
the majority of it would be converted into fat once in the body and
that you would be one more step closer to injecting yourself with
insulin, seems to be neither here nor there for the 'fat free' industry.
After all, your health is not their real concern, they're after what's in
your pocket.

Since the late 1970s the percentage of fat consumption per head
has decreased by about 16 per cent – that's *decreased*, gone down,

reduced. Yet obesity has doubled since that time, with an increase in the average weight of 12lb. *So we are fatter now than we were when we were eating more fat.* The only foodstuffs whose consumption has increased in exact correlation to how fat we are getting is WHITE REFINED SUGAR AND CARBS – coincidence? Make up your own mind. These facts illustrate just how meaningless these 'low fat' and 'fat free' labels are, especially as the manufacturers tend to add more sugar in place of the fat.

The wording they use to lure people into buying these products is often pretty deceptive too. If you saw two packets of biscuits on a shelf, one is '80 per cent fat free' and the other contains 20 per cent fat, which one would you be more likely to buy? The truth is that so many more people would choose the apparent 'fat free' version, even though both packets contain exactly the same amount of fat. Or maybe they do, the truth is you never really know the true fat content anyway. I had an expert on this particular subject explain that if you take the calorie blah blah and times it by the what-do-ya-call-it and then divide it by how many who-do-ya-ma-flips there are, the true fat content would be revealed. But once again WE DON'T NEED TO KNOW. All we need to know is that 'fat free' and 'low fat' is often a huge lie and most of the time it usually means that more white refined sugar and salt have been added to improve the taste. The salt content alone causes water retention, again adding weight and totally defeating said purpose. It also helps to push your blood pressure sky high. Yes there really is nothing like a good low fat food to keep you slim and healthy. And the 'fat free' products I am talking about are literally *nothing* like a good low fat food.

POTATOES ARE FOR PIGS, CORN IS FOR CATTLE

And whilst I am on the subject of 'low fat' or 'fat free' foods, here's another eye opener. Baked potatoes – the very product we turn to when trying to lose weight – can cause your sugar levels to rise and a massive amount of insulin to be released. And, just to make sure by the end of the book you really know this stuff, don't forget insulin is the *fat-producing* hormone. Insulin in the bloodstream also prevents stored fat from being broken down – double whammy. Not only does it store fat, it also inhibits the fat it stores from being broken down – bugger! Am I saying don't eat potatoes? No. Am I saying that potatoes are as bad as a Mars Bar? No! Am I saying that potatoes contain no vitamins, minerals or essential fibre? No – this is not Fatkins remember (oh sorry, I mean Atkins). All I'm saying is that if weight loss is a concern for you, no longer be deluded into thinking baked potatoes are the good slimming food we believe them to be.

POP GOES ANOTHER THEORY

Popcorn is another apparent 'low fat' food. But once again corn causes insulin release and boom, the same problem. Popcorn is usually covered in sugar anyway, so the insulin problem is compounded. And those of you who go for the salt option aren't missing out either – the corn itself shoots the sugar levels sky high while the salt shoots the blood pressure sky high. The French have always said, 'Potatoes are for pigs and corn is for cattle'. Why? Because they help to fatten them up. How many times have we avoided smearing butter on our potatoes or corn on the cob, yet it's the corn and potatoes which are largely responsible for the weight gain, rather than the butter. I know that it's not easy to change a belief, especially about potatoes or corn, but I did ask you to read this stuff with an open mind.

'If you can pinch more than an inch, you should go on a diet'

Do you remember the advert? Do you remember what they were advertising? 'Special K' – a white refined carbo breakfast, which was labelled 'low fat' and in fact still is all these years later. I believe the catchphrase used in that advert caused more people to believe they had a weight problem than any other in history. In my opinion it caused many people to unnecessarily start dieting. And as we now know, dieting makes you fat. What did they mean if you *can* pinch more than an inch? It should have been 'If you *can't* pinch more than an inch, then you're in big trouble.' My mother recently lost her husband and, as a result, had very little appetite. She reached the stage where she *couldn't* pinch more than an inch. This is not a sign of health: when the body reaches this level it can start to eat its own organs.

The 'Special K' advert was a big part of the anti-fat campaign, which started in the '70s and has been going strong ever since. We have been bombarded with so much anti-fat propaganda over the years that we now believe there is something wrong with consuming even the good, essential fats that are needed for the body to function properly. The amount of people I get in my seminars who believe avocados and olives are fattening is a joke. I am not knocking them as I used to believe this rubbish too. Two 'diet' clubs told me that avocados, nuts and olives are full of fat. The fact is these diet clubs were not lying, they are full of fat, but what they fail to tell you is that they are full of *good* fats – and that is good news. The fats in these foods will *not* make you fat, they are designed by nature to give the body the essential fats it needs and craves. The body cannot produce these fats by itself, which is why they are known as *essential*. It is vital we put fat into our body, but it is equally vital that it's the right kind. Never has one food been so misunderstood by so many. Let me lay this bogie to rest once and for all: avocados will not make you fat and they don't contain cholesterol.

The average child in the UK will consume 52st (728lb) of the *wrong* kind of fat between the ages of six and 16. Can you imagine – 52 STONE OF FAT. That is the equivalent of 1,314 packets of lard. Is it any wonder children as young as eight are showing signs of heart disease? Essential fats are *not* the problem, we need them – they are not described as *essential* for nothing. It's the stuff you find bacon and egg swimming around in on a Sunday morning that's the real problem. I now get through at least three avocados a day so I think that qualifies me to state categorically that avocados will not make you fat. I don't know who was responsible for claiming that they did but for the record – CHOLESTEROL CANNOT BE FOUND IN THE PLANT KINGDOM. Animals and humans (and to a lesser extent seafood) are the only living things capable of producing cholesterol. It is therefore impossible for avocados or nuts, eaten in their *natural* state, to cause cholesterol problems. When nuts are heated, on the other hand, this damages the good oils and can cause the body to produce more of its own cholesterol in a bid to protect itself. However, the cholesterol didn't come from the nut or avocado, but was created by the body in response to a de-natured food.

So as well as eating loads of delicious avocados, I also eat quite a few nuts (in their natural state), always have oil on my salads (olive oil and occasionally flaxseed), love oily fish and eat plenty of olives. There is nothing wrong with doing this, it won't make you fat or unhealthy, despite what some 'experts' say. It is *not* eating enough fat that is more likely to make you both unhealthy and fat. Body fat is extremely important as it contains vital hormones which help to regulate the appetite. I want to repeat that:

Fat helps to regulate your appetite

It also boosts the immune system, governs our energy metabolism, is used as an emergency energy store and helps to cushion the joints and protect the muscles. It even plays a part in our sex lives as we need fat to help make hormones like estrogen and testosterone. Fat also stimulates the brain, so it is hardly surprising that very low fat diets have been linked with depression and other mental disorders.

Remember, just like the wrong kind of sugar, it's the *wrong kind* of fat which does the damage. If you keep putting in the wrong type of fats, your body will continue to crave the fat it really needs. In other words, the wrong fats create an even *greater* need for fat than necessary. The problem is when you first give yourself a 'wrong fat hit' you *will* feel better, but not for long. The body will soon realize that what it has been given is not the real stuff, and once again will send a signal to the brain saying 'I need more fat'. So you either use your willpower and control not to have any more (as you have been told *all* fat is bad) or you say 'Sod it – one doughnut won't hurt'. Either way, the body is, once again, lacking *genuine* sustenance. This creates a feeling of dissatisfaction in the body, which naturally has a knock-on effect on the mind.

One particular target of the 'anti-fat' movement was butter. Now I am not about to start saying that butter is good, because it's not. But it is certainly nowhere near as bad as the synthetic lumps of hydrogenated oil which the manufacturers claim are a 'healthy' alternative because they are made from things such as sunflower oil or olive oil.

They say these 'spreads' are 'high in polyunsaturates and low in saturates'. But, quite frankly, this is just more blah, blah, blah talk because what they fail to tell us is that in order to get the sunflower or olive oil from a liquid to a block it has to be heated. Heating the oil at a high temperature for a long time creates hydrogen bubbles, which makes the oil solidify. 'So what' you say. Unfortunately exposing oil to a high temperature completely changes its chemical structure to one which the body has a massive challenge dealing with. Put simply, the oil changes from a good fat to a bad one.

So, to sum up: it's the *wrong* type of fat and the massive amounts of white refined sugar and carbs which make people fat and unhealthy. There is nothing wrong with the good fats – so eat and enjoy.

As well as sugar, there is another white refined drug food hidden in many low fat, so-called healthier foods which people just don't seem to be too bothered about. In fact this life-shortening drug food is in virtually every processed food we buy, yet it is rarely seen as a major concern by the public. Most people are more concerned about losing weight and looking good to get hot and bothered about this substance. But it's about time we took a very realistic look at a killer substance that we are so badly hooked on that we even add tons more of the stuff to 'foods' that are already heavily laced with it. If feeling good, supreme health and long life are on your agenda then I strongly suggest you open your mind, take your head out of the sand and stop taking this subject with a very deadly...

9

Pinch of Salt

If only it were a pinch then we really wouldn't have a problem. A pinch might be all you add to your food, but what about the 220,000 tons of white refined salt that the food industry adds to its products every year in the UK alone? This stuff contains nothing of any nutritional value to the body whatsoever, it is highly addictive and it is one of the country's single biggest killers. According to a recent study, if food manufacturers cut the salt they use by half, a whopping 100,000 lives a year could be saved. But, once again, as long as this stuff doesn't kill people straight away and they have enough time to rake in some hard cash from their customers, what the hell do they care?

WE JUST HAVEN'T GOT THE HEART FOR IT

White refined table salt contains highly toxic sodium – yes toxic. Here's another load of total bull we've been fed, 'salt is good for you'. Says who? The people who make billions from the stuff? Let's get something clear – white refined salt is very, very toxic to the human body. If there is too much of it, the kidneys have to work their socks off to get rid of it. This in turn makes the heart work harder. And when the heart works harder, it pumps loads more blood through the kidneys – which means the end result is high blood pressure and high blood pressure equals strokes and heart attacks.

Despite this fact, the drug food industry hides tons of this water-retaining, high blood pressure-producing, stroke-inducing substance in 'foods' that are specially aimed at children. The advertising is also aimed at kids too. I hardly think the adverts for crisps and Mr Ronald McDonald's latest promotion are aimed and your average adult, do you? In fact 96 per cent of American children recognize Mr Ronald McDonald. To put this in perspective, the only other fictitious character who is recognized more is Santa Claus. Get them hooked whilst they're young is usually the policy of any self-respecting drug pusher and the drug food industry is no different. They seem unconcerned that children as young as four are already showing changes in their veins and arteries similar to those found in the early stages of hypertension, and that if they carry on using this substance throughout their lives they have a massive chance of either losing use of certain parts of their body through a stroke, or losing their life as a result of Britain's biggest killer – heart disease. The makers also know that if you give a child, or anyone for that matter, salty foods it will make them thirsty. In turn they sell more fizzy drinks (more about that later), which once again equals more money for the industry. That's why you see so many heavily salted snacks on bars in pubs and wine bars, it's not because they're being generous – it's to get you to buy more drink.

HIDDEN EXTRAS

A single bowl of standard cornflakes contains the same amount of salt as a whole bowl of sea water. A pizza contains about one teaspoon of salt – and that's before we sprinkle our fix over it. Even commercially-baked bread contains loads of the stuff. There are just too many foods containing artery-strangling refined salt to list them all. Not only do companies add a lot of 'hidden' salt to their foods but many encourage us to add even more. Look at the size of the average saltcellar at your local drug food outlet (better known as fast food joints) – they're huge. Each one of the holes in the top of their converted salt bucket lets out enough salt to squeeze any vein or artery into submission! And the only reason they add loads of salt and encourage us to do the same is because it is addictive and it helps them to sell more drug drinks.

One thing is for certain, you can be guaranteed that virtually every processed food you buy *already* contains salt, so you will be doing yourself a massive favour by leaving the saltcellar off the kitchen table. And this doesn't just apply to when you're eating processed foods. You do not need to add salt to natural foods either – despite what some 'experts' say. There is one simple reason –

The amount of salt we need is in the foods nature provides for us

I can only think that the experts are getting somewhat confused about the sodium and salt issue. Instead of saying refined salt is good for us, what they meant to say of course was, 'The body does need sodium, but only in its natural state – like the kind you find in foods such as fruits, green leafy vegetables, celery etc.'

At this point I can just hear you saying, 'But Jason, it tastes so good, what would a boiled egg be like without the salt?' It tastes just as good, but when I was hooked on salt I would never have believed it and at this stage I wouldn't blame you for thinking the same. But the truth is once you stop having salt on any food – i.e. you 'change your brand' – it soon starts to taste great without it. Unfortunately, salt isn't something we can realistically expect to avoid entirely as it is found in just about everything. However, once you've changed your brand of all foods you will automatically be free from most of the hidden salt found in drug and junk foods.

So why does the drug food industry love the stuff so much? It's a great preservative (so much so that the Egyptians used to use it for storing dead bodies), it causes dehydration, it's cheap and highly addictive – the perfect ingredient as far as they're concerned. And whilst I'm on the subject of 'preserving', did you know that we now consume so much salt and other preservatives in our food that are bodies are no longer decomposing when we die? How wonderful.

There are, of course, many people who know all about good fats and bad fats and about the harmful effects of white refined sugar and salt;

there are also many who can see behind some of this advertising nonsense, but despite this, they still continue to consume these 'foods'. I know this first hand, because I was one of them. At the time I didn't know all of the bad things sugar does, but even if I had that knowledge it wouldn't have stopped me. Why? Because I thought at the time that I totally loved my old brand and that there was just no pleasure in consuming anything else. I thought I might have a slightly shorter life, but so what. At least it will be fun and not dull and boring. I don't want to turn into one of those health freaks thank you very much. I may be fat, but at least I'm happy. At least I get pleasure from what I eat. At the same time we all use the infamous 'Uncle Fred' story to justify our apparent genuine 'choice'. The problem is the longer you told the Uncle Fred story, the older he became and more junk he consumed. In the end, Uncle Fred drank a bottle of Scotch a day, ate nothing but fry-ups, smoked 100 cigarettes a day, lived till he was 650 and of course *never* had a day's illness in his entire life. Sadly, we not only end up believing anything we tell ourselves over and over again, but we regard Uncle Fred as some kind of genuine market research and ignore the enormous number of people who are having their lives cut short because of what they are putting inside their bodies.

The sad reality is that many people whose health has deteriorated to the point where they have been told to literally diet or die, still continue to eat and drink themselves to death. Smokers know that cigarettes are likely to kill them, but still continue to smoke, even when they have had a leg amputated. Why? Because although people know they *could* die *someday* from smoking or eating rubbish, they also believe there is a genuine pleasure in doing it and they literally fear life without it. All drug addicts want to stop taking their drug, given the genuine choice, but all drug addicts want to continue taking their drug too. The nature of drug addiction is a mental tug of war caused by an illusionary belief about what the addict perceives they get from the drug. The same principle applies to drug food addiction. This tug of war in the mind cannot be removed by simply sticking a patch on, eliminating the wrong foods, taking slimming tablets, having your stomach stapled, or eating nothing but cabbage for three weeks. These only treat the *physical* symptoms of something that has a *psychological* cause. The problem can only be eliminated by removing the many years of brainwashing and conditioning and coming to a full understanding of the nature of drug foods.

As I will repeatedly stress throughout this book, the real problem people have when attempting to change their eating habits is not physical. The physical feelings of emptiness that occur as a result of things like caffeine withdrawal or low blood sugar take days to get over. In many cases, the feelings are so slight you won't even notice them anyway – especially when you start to furnish your body with the right stuff. How many times have you felt really hungry but for some reason you got involved with something else? In other words you changed your mental focus. You go for hours doing whatever it is that has taken your mind off the hunger, but what *physical* pain are you in? None whatsoever. Once you remember that you haven't eaten you will then eat. But the minute you go on a diet you are hungry all of the time – why? Because you are simply *mentally* hungry for the pleasure you believe you are missing out on. And this is what the problem amounts to – a self-imposed mental tantrum caused by the belief we have just had something worthwhile taken from us. But what is so worthwhile about eating junkie and drug food? Exactly how does it make us happy? What does it really do for us? What is the point in eating or drinking it? And what exactly will we be missing out on if we just decided to dump them from our lives?

It is time to explode the myth once and for all that when you change your brand of food you will be missing out on…

10

The Wonderful Pleasures of Eating Rubbish

Ah yes, the wonderful and joyous pleasures of consuming rubbish. This is where the advertising, conditioning and illusionary effects of drug-like foods really come into play. They all combine very nicely to fool us into thinking drug-like foods are simply wonderful and fruit and veg is for very boring people with long hair who live up trees. Manufacturers and advertisers use whatever they believe is pleasurable and try to link it to their product. The idea is to make us think that we will get the same genuine pleasure by eating or drinking whatever it is they are selling, while at the same time creating the illusion we can possibly avoid some pain in the process. There is one major problem with this approach – it works. They are targeting our basic human driving forces – a desire for pleasure and a need to avoid pain. On top of this false advertising we have the 'foods' or 'drinks' themselves which do *appear* to give us pleasure and take away a degree of pain; thus giving the adverts some degree of credence.

However, the fact is that unless it's an absolute emergency, there's simply nothing whatsoever to be gained from consuming rubbish foods and drinks. Now before you throw the book in the bin thinking that I have now totally lost the plot and am talking complete clap-trap, hear me out. I am not saying that you don't *feel* some degree of pleasure when you initially eat white refined drug foods or drink high-sugar fluids, because you do. What I am saying is it's a *false* pleasure based on the ending of a *false* physical and/or mental hunger caused by the 'foods' themselves and/or the advertising.

If I am feeling low due to my sugar levels crashing or a lack of the right fats (or both), there is no question that if I eat a fast food burger and fries plus a sugary drink, I am definitely going to feel better, thus get some pleasure. But the pleasure is simply the momentary ending of an aggravation. Unless I have low blood sugar to start with I am not going to get the pleasure. But who in their right mind would deliberately cause their sugar levels to drop to a dangerous level and create a completely unnecessary false hunger simply in order to get the 'pleasure' of ending it? That would be the same as deliberately listening to say Des O'Connor sing simply in order to get the pleasure and relief of turning him off!

The ending of an aggravation is pleasurable – but why deliberately cause the aggro in the first place?

The ending of these false physical hungers is far from the only thing to create this illusion of genuine pleasure. We have the advertisers constantly creating a host of illusions on our TV screens to lure us to their apparent irresistible pleasure – to try and back up the *initial* feeling we get when we consume their rubbish. And the biggest pleasure they use to peddle their wares is sex. And let's face it – sex sells. The drug food industry uses it at every available opportunity. Just picture the very attractive lady lying in that beautiful claw-bath, water overflowing onto the floor of a huge luxurious bathroom. Slowly, seductively, sexually, eating a chocolate bar to the tune of 'Only the crumbliest, flakiest chocolate tastes like chocolate never tasted before'. Or what about the attractive woman taking a bite of a Bounty bar followed by an image of a tall, dark, handsome man smiling at her on a deserted beach (no doubt about to take her to 'paradise'). Ice cream makers have always been huge fans of linking sex with their product, just look at the Magnum and Häagen-Dazs ads. And while we are on the subject of pleasure, sex and drug-like substances, let's not forget the Diet Coke man and his 11.30 Diet Coke break. I think the fact that they're using sex to sell this product is pretty undisputed. What the advert is saying is this: if you're a man and you drink Diet Coke you will look like the window cleaner in the ad and all women, just like those in the ad, will want to sleep with you. If you're a woman, it's saying if you drink Diet Coke you'll get to sleep with men who look like the hunky window cleaner. So it's totally true to life then!

These ads and hundreds of thousands like them use either sex or some type of emotional pleasure trigger to help sell their 'stuff'. However, what on earth have any of the images we see in these type of ads got to do with the so-called foodstuffs they're advertising? NOTHING WHATSOEVER. The substance being sold in the Diet Coke ad does not solve weight problems; in fact there are many reports that suggest these sorts of drinks cause you to *gain* weight. Such diet drinks are simply designed to make people *believe* they are doing something good. But do we really ever believe it? I used to go into a burger joint and order a flipple dipple whopple dopper burger, two large fries, an apple pie and of course – a *Diet* Coke. Who was I kidding? Not only that, but there is a substance in all diet drinks which scientists now believe causes overeating (more on this later).

Look at the flake ad. I don't know about you but lying in a hot bubble bath, in the middle of a luxurious bathroom, without a care in the world I should well imagine is very pleasurable. It is a pleasurable *situation*. But what the hell has that got to do with a chocolate bar? They are trying to imply that the situation this lady finds herself in is pleasurable *because* of the 'flake' and has nothing to do with the amazing bathroom, the hot bubbly water, obvious wealth and an incredible lifestyle. NO – it's the flake!

In order to break free from the food trap we must get the thought out of our minds that situations are that much more pleasurable if we are eating junk and drug foods at the same time – they aren't. I used to think that having a meal in a restaurant with friends just wouldn't be the same without a dessert. But again, how on earth does a dessert help to improve an evening with friends? Smokers believe that a meal isn't the same without a cigarette as a dessert. The dessert is just a bell, created by images and advertising in our own mind. The dessert gets *linked* to a good time, and so takes some of the credit. But the dessert doesn't *make* the good time, and this is where I got it so wrong for so long. If drug and junk foods gave us tons of genuine pleasure, if it really were the thing that made us happy, we would never need to go out. We could just sit indoors eating and eating, getting more and more pleasure, and feeling better and better. But does this happen? Not quite. I know some people do stay in and eat and eat, but they are not happy doing this, they always feel mentally and physically low afterwards. That is not genuine pleasure – it's a waste of precious life.

Genuine pleasure is where you look forward with anticipation to what you are going to do, you love it whilst you are doing it and you love the feeling of fulfilment afterwards. In other words it satisfies your needs – whatever they are. Ending a *genuine* hunger does precisely this if your need is for nutrients/fuel. That's why I now love my food, love feeling hungry and adore eating. I love the anticipation of good food, I love it whilst I am eating it and I love the feeling of total satisfaction afterwards.

When it comes to the pleasure of drug-like foods it's all about image, about creating a false need. Whatever the ad, they are selling a pleasurable *situation*, like having a hot bath in luxurious surroundings for example, and linking it to their product. And they are also selling a lifestyle. Somehow I just don't think the flake ad would have had the same impact if the bath was one of those stuck in the corner of a very small bathroom in a council flat and the woman getting into it was 20st in weight. Is it possible that your image of the flake would have been different if it were? How many would they have sold then? Imagine the window cleaner in the Diet Coke ad with a huge beer gut, builder's bum and a pair of bifocals on; all the women with bums the size of the Napa valley, dribbling over their birds-eye view of *his* amazing breasts. Once again do you think our image of these products would be different to what they are? Slightly.

HOOKED ON AN ILLUSION

These adverts are selling two illusions of pleasure. One is the image portrayed on screen; the other is the physical reaction you feel when you *first* put these drug-like foods into your body. The truth is, no matter how much these drug-like foods are dressed up, they never quite live up to our expectations. I used to always love the *idea* of eating rubbish foods, but the reality was never quite what I had in mind. This is because often what I had in my mind had actually been subconsciously planted there by some external image I had seen.

We are far from blameless when it comes to advertising either – we do it to ourselves. We often help the advertisers by creating images of wonderful situations in our mind, then we link some junk or drug food to it. Images such as vegging out watching a video with a tub of ice cream; eating a pizza whilst playing a board game with friends; or joining your friends for a dessert. But these situations are not enhanced by the foods.

Let me ask you a question. Have you ever been eating ice cream whilst watching a video and been happy at the same time? Yes, I should imagine is the answer. But have you also ever been watching a video whilst eating ice cream and been bored and miserable? Again I imagine the answer is yes. So what's changed? The ice cream is still the same, it's the particular video and how you are looking at your world that causes your feelings to change – not the ice cream. The situation is not suddenly transformed because you've had some ice cream.

Ice cream, pizza, fast foods, chocolates, cola, etc. do not make us happy – *situations* and certain people all help to make us happy. It's just that when people are *forced* to be without these things (i.e. when they're on a diet) they're so bloody miserable. The conclusion therefore is miserable without, happier with. Many overweight people say, 'I like eating this way. I'm happy eating this way. I'm fat and I'm happy'. What they really mean is I am happier than when I'm on a diet – and, yes, they are, because diets can be living hell. But these people are still nowhere near as happy as someone who is physically and mentally vibrant, slim and energy driven; who's happy with the way they look and feel; who is free to eat what they really want – someone who is in true control of their thoughts when it comes to food. Such people are not constantly thinking about what they should or shouldn't eat, they don't have to exercise control and discipline over their food intake on a daily basis: they are totally free from the food trap.

We so often bang on about how much we enjoy eating or drinking trashy foods and how we could never cope without them, yet we often feel lousy after we've eaten them and are having difficulty coping with our lives because of them. The truth is we don't really enjoy the *overall* mental and physical feelings of consuming this type of food, which is why you are reading this book. We only like the idea, the illusion – what we believe we will get from having it and, of course, the initial sugar 'hit' which creates a huge part of the illusion.

I did not enjoy being overweight, constantly tired and hating the way I looked and felt. I did not have fun waking up every morning with a trash-food hangover (more about that later). I did not feel joy trying to exercise control over what I ate every day. It did not feel good feeling bloated and guilty after I'd got fed up, said 'sod it' and indulged. I felt no great ecstasy in not being able to wear what I wanted. And I certainly didn't feel any kind of euphoria the time I ran off crying from a school football game. The teacher had forgotten the bibs, which meant one team had to go 'skins' and the other 'tops'. No problem for my thin teammates – but hell for me. I pleaded to go with the 'tops', but was ordered to 'stop being so stupid and just take your top off'. At 11 years of age, with everyone staring at me, it was just too much so off I went. I felt so down and miserable I needed comforting – I know, how about a 'happy meal' to cheer me up!

This is not pleasure, it's a nightmare. A nightmare that the 'wonderful' drug-like foods created in the first place.

'Yes Jason but what about the wonderful taste? You cannot tell me I don't like the taste of these foods, because I do.'

I know you do, I am not saying you don't. But do you honestly believe you put up with all you do simply because you like the taste? Do you honestly believe that people who suffer heart attacks, strokes, diabetes, the constant disability of being overweight because of their food addictions do so because it's the taste that they couldn't resist? Or are you now starting to realize it's all just part of the subtle food trap?: that it's a physiological compulsion created by a false physical hunger and a thousand different images we've seen over the years. It really is not about taste. I used to have a compulsion to smoke cigarettes, but was the compulsion due to the wonderful taste of cigarettes? I never ate one of them! No, I was mentally hooked on what I *thought* a cigarette did for me and I was fearful of letting go. I felt insecure because of the cigarettes yet they *appeared* to make me feel more secure – it was a loop. And the same applies here. We just are more easily fooled with sugar because it tastes sweet, we naturally have a sweet tooth and everyone around us thinks it's normal.

If I gave you a hamburger and fries, which to you tasted absolutely delicious, and as you were eating them I told you the burger was made from dead cockroaches found on the kitchen floor, and the fries were in fact dried up crushed toenail clippings with added salt, would you carry on eating eat them? No, neither would I – no matter how wonderful they tasted. In those circumstances you can keep the taste thank you very much.

People caught in the food trap are not hooked on the taste; they may believe they are, as it seems the only rational reason. They are hooked on a belief, an idea, a set of images and illusions set up to trap them. This is why it is so easy to escape from the food trap – you are only hooked on what you *believe* you get from these foods. You are, in a sense, your own jailer. Once you realize it's all complete nonsense and follow my mental and physical recipe (the route out) – you will feel totally free.

FLAVOUR OF THE MONTH

I now honestly don't give a flying... if a burger, fries and a can of cola tastes like the seven wonders of the world, they contain white refined trash and have been chemically flavoured with God knows what, so they are bound to. But as far as I'm concerned this is worse than if they had made it from dead cockroaches and crushed toenails. Drug foods can control people's lives on a daily basis and can cause premature death. The way I used to feel and the way I feel now is just not worth the split-second taste – especially as I have changed my brand and now actually much prefer the taste of the finest fruits, salads, wholemeal breads and pastas, fresh fish and gorgeous, freshly-made fruit and vegetable juices. I get more pleasure from eating and drinking now than ever before. The taste of my food is in a different league to what it used to be. This is largely due to the fact I am now genuinely hungry every time I eat. And if you are, the pleasure of eating goes up by 1000 per cent. This is why I now have no desire to pick in-between meals. Firstly, I no longer experience false mental or physical hungers, and secondly what would be the point? If you pick you miss the very thing you think you will be deprived of – the real joy of eating.

The real joy of eating comes only when you are genuinely hungry. This enhances the taste and smell to a completely different level. A friend of mine, Brian (yes hello my Israeli friend), used to hold a lot of barbecues. I was told they were not to be missed as the food was brilliant. I arrived at 2pm fully expecting food to be served at about 4pm. I waited and waited and waited but after one thing or another, we ended up eating at 9.30pm! And guess what – it was delicious. It was bound to be because everyone was so genuinely hungry.

There is real pleasure in ending a *genuine* hunger – this totally satisfies the mind and body. There is false, short-term illusory pleasure in trying to end a *false* physical and mental hunger – and it creates long-term pain.

The short and long-term pain these types of food create becomes part of the loop. The first thing I did when I felt down or depressed was head straight for the fridge. If I ate what was in the fridge I was bound to feel depressed and down. So I would carry on with what I call the ultimate 'sod it' mood. 'I've started so what the hell, I've done it now, I may as well just carry on.' But why did I head for the fridge in the first place? I wasn't physically hungry. I used to head for the fridge when I felt down for one reason – I honestly thought, whether consciously or sub-consciously, that I could change the way I felt by eating some food. And all the advertisers are constantly perpetuating this belief. They really do give the impression that you can...

11

Change Your Mood by Eating Some Food

We are the only creatures on the planet who eat food to try to change the way we feel. This would be fine if it worked, but it doesn't. Have you ever been bored, angry, upset, restless, or stressed at the same time as eating something? Of course, I know I have, but food cannot solve these external psychological emotions. It's the idea that our woes will be lessened by shoving something down our throat that keeps us doing it. The reality is that doing it achieves the complete opposite.

If you try and feed any kind of emotion with any type of food you will, of course, create problems. This is because the body neither wants nor needs food at these times. Usually – depending obviously on the person – whatever you eat when you are not genuinely physically hungry will be stored as fat. I want to repeat that:

Whatever you eat when you are not genuinely physically hungry will be stored as fat

It was always meant to – it's the body's incredible survival mechanism kicking in. It assumes you are loading up on food, not because you are stressed or bored, but because you sense lean times ahead and have no choice. And if there is going to be a shortage soon, the body wants to make certain it's going to survive and so stores the excess food in new, specially-made, fat cells. This principle applies even if it's natural foods but, having said that, how many people reach for natural food when trying to feed an emotion? I mean when was the last time you heard anyone saying, 'I'm really pissed off, sod it, I'm going to treat myself to a bunch of grapes' ? Not in this lifetime that's for sure.

People who eat to try to feed an emotion don't usually reach for grapes or strawberries; they reach for chocolate, cakes, fast foods and ice cream. Why? Because these are *drug*-like foods and as such people try to use them in exactly the same way as a drug addict attempts to use their drug. At the same time – on adverts, films, TV shows and in everyday life – we see other people doing it. You don't see people like Rachel from *Friends* trying to comfort herself with a bowl of cherries, do you? No, she has a big bag of crisps or a tub of ice cream to help drown her sorrows. We think, 'if it helps Jennifer, it'll help me'. But does it – NO.

EMPTY PROMISES

When you experience normal, genuine hunger there is a part of you that feels empty and slightly insecure. The same applies with the false hungers that drug-like foods create. They are designed to make a part of you feel empty. And this is why we get fooled and why we attempt to feed an emotion with drug-like food: the internal feelings we get when we are bored, stressed, lonely, down or stressed, are also empty insecure feelings, almost identical to the feelings of false and genuine hunger. When we are bored, a part of us feels empty. It's the same when we are stressed, lonely, or need comforting – a part of us feels a void, an emptiness of some kind. This feels very similar to hunger.

Now let's assume you are not genuinely physically hungry, but you are feeling down about something. If you eat loads of food are you really going to feel better about what is getting you down? No way! In fact you are guaranteed to feel worse, both mentally and physically. All that happens is the excess food is shipped into fat cells for storage – it will do nothing to help your emotion because *you cannot feed an emotion with food*. You would only feel better if genuine hunger was causing you to feel down or irritable. Then, of course, you would be 'lifted', both mentally and physically, by feeding a genuine hunger. It would genuinely solve *that* particular problem, but food of any description is incapable of solving any problem other than genuine hunger.

The irony is that eating the wrong kind of food helps to cause the change in your mood

Many people are aware that food cannot change an emotion, yet they still reach for trashy foods when feeling down. However, halfway through eating whatever it is they are using to try and 'feed' their emotion, they will feel even worse than they did, wonder why on earth they are doing it, and want to turn the clock back to the point just before they ate it. I know I did on many occasions. The problem is that *initially* – for the first couple of bites at least – drug food addicts *do* feel better than they did a moment previous. Why is this? Partly because they have told themselves they will feel better with some food. If I told myself I would feel better if I had a beach-ball and I honestly believed it would be of benefit, then in the moment someone handed it to me, as strange as it may seem, I would actually feel better – for a second at least. It's a bit like the security blanket for a child; the blanket doesn't make them feel better, they just feel mentally low when it's taken away. The reason for this is a belief about what it represents.

However, the main reason why the drug food addict feels better *initially* is because often they are either withdrawing from certain drug foods or drinks, or their blood sugar levels are out of sorts because of them. Now there is no way the drug food addict is aware of this, because they are so used to these feelings that they believe this is a normal way to feel. In addition, these feelings are identical to those of normal hunger, apprehension and stress. So if they feel stressed, lonely, bored or whatever *on top* of the empty feelings of withdrawal or low blood sugar then they're in double trouble. They will always feel worse than if this wasn't going on; their emptiness will always feel greater. But all the empty feelings get mixed up together and seem like one big one. So the minute you inject yourself with a shot of drug food or drink – which takes no digestion and just gets sucked through the stomach lining, loading the bloodstream with excess sugar – the overall empty feeling *decreases*, giving you what you believe to be, and what feels like, an instant 'hit' – instant relief from some of the emptiness you felt. So in that second you have tricked your brain and nervous system into believing that these foods help to take the edge off some kind of genuine emotion. But the edge was only there because of the trashy foods in the first place. This is why people reach for food when what they're feeling has nothing to do with genuine hunger.

BOREDOM

People often say boredom is a major cause of why they overeat. Again I used to be the first to say this. But this excuse would never wash in the wild. Imagine you see a very large overweight squirrel stuffing nut after nut into its mouth and ask it 'Why are you doing that?' Now imagine it giving the answer 'I'm bored out of my head! I've been in the same park for bloody years, seeing the same people every day. There's nothing else to do apart from eat. It fills the day.' What would you think? That's right, 'Stone me a talking squirrel!' The point is this scenario sounds so stupid because you would never see a squirrel, or any other wild animal for that matter, eating for any reason other than hunger. If you could speak animal language and asked any wild animal why were they eating they would all say, 'Because I'm hungry and I need to survive'. Ask the average human the same question and they can come up with a billion excuses, not rational reasons. After all the only rational reason is to end a genuine hunger.

I watched a documentary some time ago on attitudes to eating in different cultures. They asked one 12-year-old boy from the East, 'Why are you eating rice and vegetables?' He replied, 'Good for the heart, good for the mind and good for the soul'. Wow and he was only twelve. They then asked a 12-year-old kid from the States why he was eating a hamburger and fries: his reply was 'Hell man, it's twelve o'clock'.

I no longer care what the clock says. If I am not hungry why should I eat just because I have been conditioned to eat at certain times? If I go dancing for hours late at night I will sweat and build up an appetite, so I'll eat. I don't care who says you shouldn't eat at 3am. If I am genuinely hungry at 3am I will eat.

In order to be slim for life we have to honest with ourselves. If you are sitting indoors by yourself and you're bored out of your head, the situation will not alter if you have a chocolate bar in your hand – you will still be bored. When I was a child and I was bored, my mother would never say 'Oh, go and stuff your face, that will solve your boredom', she would say, 'go and do something'. Why did this always work? Because boredom is caused by an emptiness in your life, a momentary void whilst you think of something to do. Boredom itself is not the *cause* of why people overeat or eat the wrong types of foods. Neither is stress, loneliness or depression. The cause is the *belief* that you can dispel negative emotions with food. Without that belief you won't eat when you bored, stressed, lonely or depressed. For the same reason you would probably never take heroin when you're stressed or bored. For not only do you know it would *not* solve the problem, you are well aware it would result in a living nightmare. The fact is many people are going through a living nightmare every day because of drug-like foods.

If you are bored it is not a sign you are low on chocolate or that you have a burger and fries deficiency. It simply means you need to do something. Instead of eating you need to look for something that will genuinely fill these moments. If food really did solve boredom it would certainly solve the school holiday problem. No need to try and keep them entertained for six weeks, just let them stuff their faces. If it really did solve depression, no one would be depressed; they would just eat and be happy. If you are stressed or lonely you need to accept that you are not low on ice cream or chocolate, therefore they will not solve the problem.

The truth is not only do these foods fail to do what we think, but they do the complete opposite. They are often the very reason why you feel bored, tired, stressed and in the mood where you can't be bothered to do anything. The irony is we attempt to use this type of food to improve our mood, yet often our mood is a direct result of the food itself. When I used to smoke I would say, 'I smoke because I'm stressed' – it never dawned on me that I was stressed because I smoked.

The point is this – white refined trash affects the central nervous system causing feelings of irritability, restlessness, low blood sugar and emptiness. It puts stress on every organ in the body and helps to speed up the ageing process. The wrong type of fats clog up the arteries, cause blood cells to literally stick together and they starve the body of its life force – oxygen. There is no question that this will affect the way you feel on a *daily* basis. Just look at the many children you see in the supermarket screaming for their next sugar fix and tell me drug foods don't affect human behaviour. And let's not forget the effect of the 'E' numbers that are added to so many processed foods.

ON ONE MATEY

Ever heard the expression 'Are you on one matey?' Well, it's a question often asked in clubs in reference to the drug Ecstasy – commonly known as just 'E'. But these aren't the 'E's I'm interested in. I'm talking about the many 'E' numbers found in products masquerading as 'foods'. These apparently harmless additives are anything but. The next time you see a child, or adult for that matter, acting hyper or strangely it may be worth asking them, 'Are you on one matey?' But which one? E102 perhaps, otherwise known as tartrazine, which is used in breadcrumbs to coat things like fish fingers and the like and has been closely linked to asthma and hyperactivity. Or how about E110 (Sunset Yellow FCF), a beautiful colouring used in many children's drinks, which has been linked to asthma and also eczema. Then it could be E220, which is no less than sulphur dioxide; or the little beauty E252 (potassium nitrate) which is no less than a fertilizer. Oh and let's not forget that they could be on ethylene bisdithiocarba-mate, a fungicide used on potatoes and one which causes tumours and birth defects in laboratory animals. Is it possible that putting these things into the human body along with the sugars and salts, may affect the way we think and behave? It's not just *possible* – IT'S A FACT.

One deputy head teacher, Cherry Lazenby, completely banned sweets and fizzy drinks during break times at school because the children were becoming difficult to control and teach.

'Immediately after morning break and lunchtimes there is a difference in the children's behaviour. They are hyper, noisy, rowdy, and can't sit still or concentrate.' She goes on to say, 'Surveys have revealed that many pupils eat vast quantities of food with a high sugar content and with additives known to contribute to hyperactivity'. But again you don't need surveys or scientific research, just have a look you around at people's behaviour.

ANOTHER DOSE OF HYPERACTIVE DRUG FOOD

Yet despite growing evidence, people still don't seem willing to see the clear link between certain foods and behaviour. Children with ADHD (Attention Deficit Hyperactive Disorder), for instance, are being given drugs like Ritalin to try and calm them down – the problem is nothing to do with that can of soda, chocolate, crisps, E numbers etc., oh no the child is clearly low on Ritalin. This drug is described as the 'chemical cosh' because of its ability to 'calm' hyper children. But it is said by many parents to simply turn their kids into zombies. You could inject some anesthetic into the kids and get pretty much the same effect – but what does it do to treat the *cause*? I am not saying that *all* ADHD is caused by foods, but there is just no question that when you consume foods that create all kinds of problems for the natural balance of the body it is going to have an impact on the natural balance of the mind.

How exactly does junk and drug food help to cheer you up? How exactly does it help to relieve boredom? How exactly does it help to lessen your stress? It is stressful not being able to wear what you want, when you want. It is upsetting hating the way you look and feel on a daily basis. It is horrible to have people staring at you, judging you. It is stressful not having the energy to really enjoy what life has to offer. And it's incredibly stressful constantly having to exercise control over food – trying not to have too much, or feeling down because you have. How exactly does this rubbish help to lessen your stress? It doesn't. The truth is it does the complete opposite – and to think I used to actually fear what life would be like if I made the change. There was and is nothing to fear; I love it here and I certainly have no intention of ever going back.

YOU'RE OFF TO MAURITIUS

I see it as the North Peckham estate vs. Mauritius. What the hell am I on about? When I was overweight, constantly tired, lethargic, badly asthmatic and covered from head to toe in psoriasis, it was like constantly living on the North Peckham estate. Now for those of you who have never heard of this place, it was like mini Beirut – a good place to drive through on your way to somewhere nice! I lived on the estate for a year – not good. Whilst I was in living there *everything* in my life was more stressful. Did I ever have any good times whilst living there? Yes of course, but not because I was there, *in spite* of the fact I was there. I equate this with when I was overweight – I had some great times then too, but those times would have been just so much better if I had been slim and mentally free from the food trap. The way I feel now is like living in Mauritius. I have never actually been to the place, but it's what I imagine it to be. A bad day in Mauritius is better than the best day on the North Peckham estate. It's just a different world. The food and drinks are so much better here. They taste so wonderful that I want to take my time eating and drinking them just to savour the flavours. When I was in North Peckham I used to just scoff the food down. The foods and drinks here even contain things that boost my energy levels, which is good because there is so much to do here! I seem to get along with people better than I did. I feel awake and so alive in the mornings here. My breathing is so much better and I am a million times happier than I was.

The excellent news is it really is very easy to get to Mauritius and this is why you can start to get excited already. When I say in my seminars that someone's food/weight problem can be solved in just one day, many people think it impossible. This is because people think a weight problem will take months to solve, depending on how much *physical* weight they have to lose. But the problem is how people look at food, what they think it does for them. Before you put anything into your mouth you must think first. Once people change the way they see foods, their problem is already solved. It took me over six months to arrive safe and sound in Mauritius, but I loved the journey. The minute I boarded the plane I knew my problem was solved.

You have so much to look forward to, but before you even think of boarding the plane all the brainwashing and conditioning must be removed. This is why I urge you to FINISH THIS BOOK; don't think you're ready for the trip yet. If you start now you'll find the take-off fine, but you'll inevitably crash. I have not yet given you one single ingredient for my recipe for success. The recipe is essential, but before I share it with you we need to look at *all* the problematic foods and drinks in depth. In terms of what you are going to achieve this won't take that long, but please understand that the 'how to' part only comes in the last quarter, so please finish the entire book. Finishing the book and following the correct thought process enables you to fly first class and guarantees a safe landing in the beautiful world of Mauritius. *Not* reading the whole book guarantees a life in the North Peckham estate. The choice is yours, but having reaped the amazing life-changing benefits myself I urge to do what over 90 per cent of people who buy a book of this nature fail to do, which is to actually finish reading it.

I think I've made my point, so let us continue our journey with perhaps the most reached-for drug-like food in times of emotional need. It is arguably one of the most falsely advertised drug-like foods out there – a product that people have been totally conditioned to believe will change the way they feel: a real mood food. If you really want success, it's time to say...

12

Chocs Away!

First of all, before we get into all the conditioning, advertising and misinformation that surrounds this stuff, let's just look at what it is. Chocolate does not naturally grow on trees, it is a man-made substance. People sometimes argue that cocoa (one of the main ingredients of chocolate) is natural, but you could carry that way of thinking as far as you like – after all heroin is natural and so too is tobacco.

Have you ever actually tasted unsweetened cocoa? Take my word for it, it tastes disgusting. What makes it taste so disgusting is a drug-like substance called theobromine, which is contained in all chocolate: the darker the chocolate the more it contains. Theobromine, like any drug, causes a need for more and more. This is why when you think about having 'just the one' you will continue to eat, even if you start to feel bloated and sick. Obviously, this isn't good for you but it's excellent for the manufacturers.

Theobromine tastes disgusting, so how on earth did they ever get so many people to eat this stuff? Easy, just add good old white trashy sugar of course – backed up, once again, by massive advertising. The sugar not only gives a hit of pure glucose to the bloodstream, but it covers up the taste of the theobromine. Don't forget if you did taste it, you wouldn't eat it. But they want you to eat it, because it compels you to eat more. So now when you eat it you end two false hungers at once, wow double the pleasure. Again – not quite. That's like putting on Max Bygraves *and* Des O'Connor at the same time and getting the double pleasure of turning them both off. But again, why put them on in the first place?

What else do we find in many chocolate bars apart from these two poisonous drug-like substances? Hydrogenated vegetable fat, skimmed milk powder, fat-reduced cocoa milk, fat, malt extract, full cream milk powder, salt, lactose, whey powder, egg white, milk protein, flavouring, biscuit, yeast, crisped cereal, colourings (E171, E120, E101, E160, E133), glazing agents, butterfat, lecithin – plus many more I have undoubtedly missed.

Now a lot of that is blah, blah, blah talk. But hydrogenated oil is something to be aware of. You may not see 'hydrogenated fat/oil' on the label of some mass-market chocolate bars – instead they may put the less threatening 'trans-fatty acids'. But if the name is less threatening it doesn't make the fat any less so. For years the harmful effects of this type of oil have been common knowledge to the people in the know. Hydrogenated oil or 'trans-fat' can easily create a build-up of LDL cholesterol (the bad one), the small LDL molecules squeezing beneath the blood vessel linings, narrowing the passageways with a layer of 'plaque'. The process of hydrogenating fats creates molecules which are forced into shapes that were never designed to fit in the human body and they have been found to be a *major* cause of heart disease and cancer. In fact, just so we know what we're dealing with here, this kind of fat is so harmful that US government experts have declared *'there is no safe level of consumption'*. In light of this Mars and Nestle made newspaper headlines in 2003 when they announced to the British people they were removing 'trans-fats' from *some* of their chocolate bars. But, please don't be deluded into thinking that whatever replacement fat they have in mind will be health in a wrapper. Always remember it took many years before trans-fats were seen in their true light, so don't be surprised if the replacement fat hits the headlines at some point in the future.

Then, of course, we have the milk products. One chocolate bar manufacturer even bragged 'A pint and a half of pure cream milk goes into every bar'. A few years ago I would have thought that was good, but that was in the days when I thought for some reason we had the same digestive system as a calf! Am I now suggesting that milk is a drug-like food? No. But it is a junk food, which I will cover in depth very soon. This means you do not have to eliminate it completely from your diet, but after you have read the chapter on milk, I can almost guarantee you will want to reduce your intake drastically.

As well as the detrimental ingredients used to hook us on this stuff, we have the massive amount of advertising dedicated to promoting chocolate as a mood enhancer. They have managed to create a set of bells for virtually any occasion. Chocolate is seen as the ultimate treat and the ultimate mood food.

'A Mars a day will help you work, rest and play'

Whoever let that slogan past the advertising standards needs stringing up. It is totally false advertising. How can a Mars chocolate bar help you to work, rest and play? The ad also contradicts itself anyway. How can you rest and play? How can you work and rest? They are saying that this chocolate bar can do two complete opposites. And how on earth can it help you work? Oh yes I almost forgot, if you are eating them on a regular basis you will of course have false hungers, blood sugars crashing and all that. Those false hungers affect your concentration, so your work is affected. Once you feed them you no longer have them bugging you, thus you can now work with full concentration. But again it hasn't helped you to work, it *caused* the problem in the first place. I found out recently that someone actually took Mars to court over their 'it helps you work rest and play' slogan. Guess what? Mars won – I'd love to know how they proved their slogan to be true.

Virtually every chocolate bar ad is either aimed at children (get them hooked whilst they're young), or has an emotion linked to it – a way of supposedly helping you out in times of emptiness. A Bounty Bar will supposedly take you to paradise; a Twix will apparently help you escape 'the norm' (that little grey git). You can take time out with a chocolate bar that is actually named Time Out. You can also have a break with a Kit Kat or give yourself a boost with a bar called Boost, or you can be a real man with a Yorkie Bar. When I now see these ads it makes me wonder why I didn't see just how stupid they were.

The sheer audacity of some of the chocolate ads never ceases to amaze me. I recently watched an ad for an Aero bar featuring a woman sitting behind a desk, clearly bored out of her head. Looking for something to do to ease her boredom she reaches for an Aero. As soon as she takes a bite her whole face lights up, sparks fly from her mouth and a gospel choir comes out of nowhere. Everyone's clapping, smiling, happy and singing the tune of 'Why can't all chocolate feel this way'. Because of course that is precisely what happens when you eat an Aero bar isn't it? In reality, the woman would be sitting behind her desk bored out of her head, reach for the Aero and whilst eating would still be totally bored out of her head. Why? Because her problem is not caused by a lack of chocolate, therefore it will not be solved with some. She has a good job deficiency. The advertisers, however, are creating a bell on a subconscious level – and it works.

The truth is this approach has worked so well for chocolate that most people give this stuff to their friends and loved ones as a way of saying 'Thank You' or 'I love You'. Think of the Cadbury's Roses advert. It's all about people doing nice things for people and getting rewarded with this particular box of chocolates. They show this over and over again along with a catchy tune 'Thank you very much for doing the dishes, thank you very much, thank you very, very, very much'. In the end when you think of a good way of saying thank you, you will think of their product. They have managed to get people to say thank you with a product which is known to be addictive, clogs the arteries, makes people feel mentally low and contributes massively to weight gain. Thank you very much indeed.

Chocolate is now linked to so many days and times of the year: Mother's day, Father's day, Valentine's day – any day, in fact, seems like a good day. Easter to most people now simply means chocolate eggs. When I was a child, up until about the age of ten or eleven, there would always be a stocking full of delicious, wonderful-tasting fruit and nuts on the end of my bed on Christmas morning. I cannot recall exactly what year it changed, but it soon became the norm to have a stocking stuffed with chocolate. So strong is the conditioning with this stuff that some people even give it to sick people whilst they are lying in hospital. Cheers guys.

I read an article with disbelief recently in which a psychologist said, 'Eating chocolate has a calming effect and helps us deal with stress'. Her theory is based on her observation that 'people tend to feel calmer after eating chocolate and high fat meals. It is suspected that it is chocolate's combination of sweet creamy texture and high fat that makes it irresistible'. First of all, who feels calmer? Those who are suffering the irritable effects of low blood sugar? Just a thought. And what does she mean 'irresistible'? This kind of talk gives the impression that you can never break free from this substance. Of course chocolate is totally resistible and of course you can break free. If you were eating some chocolates and half way through eating them I informed you that what you were in fact eating was not chocolates but crushed cockroaches that had been sweetened with sugar, covered up with milk and chemicals, exactly how much of an overwhelming craving would you have then? How irresistible would they be then? This proves that the physical compulsion is easily laid to rest once you see things for what they are. Now I know that chocolates are not made from cockroaches, but they do contain theobromine, along with a whole host of other nightmare ingredients. Having said that a leading homeopathic practitioner was overheard at a seminar saying, 'Keeping cockroaches at bay is such a problem in some chocolate factories that by law there can be up to 6 per cent of crushed cockroaches in all chocolates. They sometimes fall unnoticed into the mixtures' – lovely! I have no idea just how true that is, and given that most chocolate factories are in reality some of the cleanest places on earth, I think the chances of finding any 'choc' roaches in your average box are pretty slim – but just the thought is enough to put you off.

COMPLETELY POTTY

Even famous children's stories are not immune to the pervasive idea that chocolate is some kind of mood enhancing food. *Charlie And The Chocolate Factory* is an obvious case but it is certainly not an isolated one. In the third Harry Potter book we see chocolate being used as a comforter; literally an aid to help you get back to normal after all your happiness has been sucked away by the evil 'Dementors'. I know this is only a story, but why couldn't the author have used some bright, delicious fruit instead? We all come into contact with our own versions of Dementors every day and the people who make chocolate want you to think that if someone or something drains your happiness it can all can be solved with a bar or box of fat-, sugar- and theobromine-loaded chocolate.

The truth is that you really are on a hiding to nothing with chocolate. What can you expect to gain from eating it? The minute you have some, you either have to have more or you have to use your control to stop yourself eating more. Either way you're on to a loser. The only way to win is to dump it from your life and feel *good* about the fact you no longer have to eat it. I would now feel upset if I *had* to eat it, and when I do see people eating it I don't long for it, I just think 'What a shame. God, if only they knew'. This isn't me being 'holier than thou', or a boring git, it's just the same as if I saw someone hitting themselves on the head with a mallet – I would just feel sorry for them.

Many people say, 'But come on Jason sometimes you have to be sociable and it is sociable to eat with people'. Yes it is and I love going out for meals. It is very sociable to eat genuine food and end a genuine hunger with genuine people. But it is not sociable to eat drug-like foods with people just to be sociable, and anyone who thinks it is is totally…

13

Out to Lunch

If you are going to have a dessert at a restaurant, what is this first thing you do? Ask anybody else if they are going to 'join you'. If everyone says no, you will use the most evocative words and images you can think of to try and tempt them. You literally become a sales person for the junk and drug food industry. 'Oh go on. You only live once. They do a mouthwatering hot fudge cake covered in fresh cream. What do you think? Changed your mind?' Sometimes those desperate for someone to join them will verbally try to bully someone into ordering some of the same. When I freed myself from 'the food trap', changed my brand and was flying club-class to Mauritius (metaphorically speaking of course) I often got this type of verbal attack: 'Oh what's wrong with you, you boring git. You used to be fun. Stop being so unsociable, lighten up'. But at what point did I stop being sociable? How did I stop being fun? All I said was I don't want a dessert! The simple truth is we feel stupid eating this stuff alone, so we always consciously or unconsciously try to get people to join us. You don't get this nonsense with peaches or sardines do you? Being sociable means 'To act in a sociable manner, mix socially with others'. By not having a dessert I did not stop being sociable. I was still acting in a sociable manner and mixing socially with others.

Does this mean I don't go out for meals with my friends any more or hold dinner parties? Of course not, in fact, far from it. I love going out for meals, especially with a group of people. Often a whole evening can be centred around the food, as it is in many different cultures. There are many cultures that take hours and hours over a meal. Guests are served small courses and gradually feed themselves in-between having a great social experience. But being sociable and ending a hunger are two separate entities. If you happen to be genuinely physically hungry and you go to dinner with a group of nice and fun people, then you have two pleasures at once. You satisfy a genuine physical hunger, which makes you feel wonderful, plus you are with your friends and therefore satisfying your need for interaction and fun.

If, however, the people you are sitting next to happen to be Mr and Mrs Dull who have come all the way from Dullsville for your lack of entertainment tonight, then all the sticky dessert in the world ain't going to make any difference – they will still be dull. Food does not make an evening, it's the people and the interaction that do.

The irony is that people who are caught in the food trap spend most of their time being unsociable because of their concerns about food. I used to avoid 'doing lunch' at times because I was trying to control my intake of food. Being fat also meant I would avoid social events such as swimming, going to the beach with friends and dancing. I was just too tired and too lethargic and often suffered from the 'I can't be bothered' syndrome. When you are on virtually any kind of diet you are completely unsociable and when you do eat you feel so lethargic you can't be bothered to be sociable.

You will be more sociable when you feel more alive, fitter and healthier. Your confidence will return to such a degree that you'll wonder how you ever managed to get by before; your nervous system will be functioning properly; your sugar levels will be balanced – and there'll be no more false hungers. You'll have more energy and you'll never feel deprived as you will have genuine freedom of choice.

On the physical side, it is incredibly easy to either shift those unwanted bulges and/or tap into a new lease of genuine energy. The truth is no one is fat – just toxic. If you carry excess weight you simply have stored poison around your body. Your body can do one of only two things with toxins: store them or get rid of them – it cannot use them. If the body does not have enough energy to get rid of them it will store them. And where does it tend to store excess waste? In fat cells. It takes energy to shift that stuff and clean you out. Your body at this time simply doesn't have the energy to do this. It spends most of its energy and time trying to digest, use and store the junk foods you are putting into your system.

As mentioned at the start of this book I read many, many books on health and nutrition, all explaining the physical side of things very well. The problem was they contradicted one another and not one single book I read ever mentioned the tremendous physical and psychological benefits of...

14

Fast Food

Yes indeed, fast food – the secret key to health, a slim body, clear skin, longevity and tremendous amounts of pure energy. Have I gone barking mad? Am I a few fries short of a seizure? Am I now suggesting, despite everything I have said, that there are tremendous health benefits in fast food? Yes, that is exactly what I am suggesting. Now before you think I am contradicting everything I have said up until now, hear me out. What I think of as *fast food* is completely different from your idea of what it is. I am not talking about junk or drug food; in fact, far from it.

The problem is that when I say *fast* food the first thing that springs to mind for most people are drug-like foods: burgers, fries, KFC, Pizza etc. That is because we talk about how fast the food gets to us. And the big fast food giants are certainly very good at getting the food to us ASAP. In fact McDonalds ran an advertising campaign in the eighties claiming if you stopped your car at traffic lights it gave you enough time to pick up a 'meal' from their 'restaurant' and be back in the car before the lights had changed. Now that is fast – super fast. But the minute this stuff hits your stomach and digestive tract it becomes *slow* food.

It slowly clogs up your arteries with fat, slowly fills your bloodstream with poisons, slowly overworks every organ in your body, slowly drains you of life, slowly stores fat, slowly speeds up the ageing process, slowly uses up valuable nerve energy, slowly seeps fat into your bloodstream, slowly causes your red blood cells to stick together, and slowly starves the cells in your body to death.

Now I would hardly describe this kind of food as fast. The only thing this type of fast food does quickly is raise the blood sugar levels, but why were they so low in the first place? And it boosts them to such an uncomfortable and abnormal level that your body has to use up some of its insulin bank account – fast. As the insulin quickly transports the excess sugars in the blood to various storage areas in the body, you soon feel the effects of low blood sugar – or a constant fast food hangover. How do you solve it? With another drug food hit to 'boost' you once again. This might come in the form of white-refined food, sugary drinks, or a caffeine 'lift' (more about coffee later).

Most fast food chains are selling drug foods. These types of food give the illusion of a 'boost' only to drag you down in no time at all after you have had them. The low you experience often feels the same as stress, boredom, loneliness or even normal hunger. It tends to be a restless state, and one that appears to be calmed with more drug foods. A clever illusion, but one that has now fooled many people for years.

And let's not forget junk food, as this food group takes tremendous nerve energy to break down, use and eliminate. Now all drug foods are also junk foods, but junk foods are not drug foods. In case this is getting a bit blah, blah, blahish, I will cover this point one more time because it is essential you know the difference. When I say junk food I mean a food that contains little or no nutrients, but one that does *not* compel you to eat more and more and one the body will get some benefit from. A drug food contains *no* live nutrients whatsoever, and does compel you to eat more –i.e. it is a food with an addictive nature. This means that although it is essential to dump drug-like foods from your life, it is not necessary to eliminate junk foods completely. However, if you want to free up energy in your body to either get rid of stored fat, or just because you want to feel light and energy driven, you need a food that is natural, nutrient packed and *fast*. When I use the expression fast food in this context, I am not talking about how fast it will get into your mouth. I'm referring to how fast will the body do three things:

digest it
extract the goodness
dispose of the leftovers

If it does all three quickly, then it is a Juice Master fast food – otherwise it's a slow, hard-to-digest drug or junk food. White refined sugar is without doubt a drug food, but it is very quickly digested. In fact it goes straight through the stomach lining without being digested. However, it falls flat on the other two fronts. The body can't extract nutrients from it because it doesn't contain any and as for the disposal of wastes, the excess is often put in long term storage as fat cells. Junk food is a little different. As you will discover in the next chapter, meat is a junk food. This means it is digested in the stomach, but it takes a long time to be digested. It also takes a long time for any nutrients to be extracted and often an eternity to dispose of the wastes. This makes junk food very *slow* food indeed, taking up valuable energy from the body that could be used for other much more worthwhile things like shifting fat, cleaning the blood, repairing damaged organs, or 'living' as opposed to 'surviving'. When it comes to junk food there is a fact you really *do* need to know:

It takes more nerve energy to digest junk food
than it does to do virtually any other activity

The average person will consume over 75 tons of food in their lifetime – that's 75 TONS! And nothing, and I do mean *no thing*, you do will ever come close to the amount of energy that's gonna be needed to deal with that huge mass of food. Oh apart from sex, which, I'm told, takes more nerve energy than anything else you can do. So now you're thinking, 'not with my partner it doesn't'. Sometimes it may not seem like it, but sex takes up a hell of a lot of nerve energy – that's my excuse for always falling asleep afterwards anyway! But yes, other than sex, it takes more energy to digest junk food than anything else you can do – including running the marathon. I realize that sounds unbelievable, but think about it. Running a marathon is tough. Twenty-six miles of sheer endurance, endeavour and incredible mental focus. If you interview someone after they have run the marathon they are of course very tired and very short of breath – but they are still awake. Try interviewing someone after they have finished a large Christmas dinner – tricky because they're usually asleep.

Do you know why people fall asleep after a big meal? There is so much junk going into the body at once that it simply doesn't have the nerve energy to cope. It then looks for every available resource of energy in order to try and break down the junk, extract whatever it can from it, get rid of whatever it can and then store what it can't get rid of (usually in fat cells). In short…

The body does not have enough energy to keep you alive and awake at the same time

This means that if you fall asleep after a big meal you are effectively in a coma. That is what happens when your body has to cut off eyesight, hearing and consciousness in order to try and muster the energy to deal with the nightmare amount of different foodstuffs that have dropped into the stomach all at once. I suppose being comatose solves the boredom problem, but it's hardly a very sociable state to be in. Oh the joys of Christmas.

Meanwhile, as you are quietly sleeping, the body is in a total 'red alert' situation; there is literally mayhem going on. Once the emergency is over the body will provide just enough energy for you to open your eyes, turn the pages of your TV guide and press the buttons on the remote control. But that's all the energy you're getting as it still has to deal with all the many courses of *slow* food you have just consumed.

Okay so Christmas dinner is a once-a-year thing, but it does illustrate the point. And if we think about it, it's not just Christmas dinner that makes us tired and sluggish. I used to often get very tired after eating a big meal in the evening, but I put it down to a hard day catching up with me and not the huge amounts of incredibly difficult-to-digest food I had consumed. But what excuse did I have for falling asleep after Sunday lunch? Was it because I was having a tough day then? The day had hardly started.

The reason I felt tired after a Sunday or Christmas lunch was because the food I had eaten was very hard for my *already* tired and battered digestive system to deal with, and so it took the energy it needed from other departments. You need to realize that every single department in the entire body will suffer in the long run if you keep doing this. If one person in a company is having to do the work load of two or three, and at the same time does not even have the correct tools to work with (i.e. live nutrients in this case), they will not be able to cope for very long and soon the whole company suffers. With all the will in the world if you have too much work for the time allocated it cannot be done and you will have to leave the work to one side (fat cells usually) in the hope that there will be some 'let up' so you can deal with it later. Your body is the same. The question is when will later be?

The human body will do anything it can to survive, despite how we abuse it. But no matter how incredible the machine, if you keep abusing it it will give up on you. Once you use up what I call your 'enzyme bank account' that's it – show's over. We are all born with a bank account of enzymes. The good news is we can add to this bank account by feeding our bodies natural, live foods which contain enzymes. The problem is drug and junk foods deplete our enzyme (life) account. So why don't we feed our bodies what they are asking for? Because our minds are being controlled by people who don't actually care if our body crumbles (as long as those selling the rubbish make their money first).

This is why it is so important to flush your mind of all the misinformation you have been subjected to about food and health, and take control of your own body. Many people look fine on the outside, but are crumbling within. What springs to mind is the seemingly 'healthy' and fit-looking 40 year old who dies of a heart attack on the tennis court. Looks are deceiving. I wonder how old his heart really was? He was 40 but his heart might have done 90 years worth of work.

If you really want a level of health and vitality you never dreamed possible, and the body of your dreams, you need to give your body a rest from this constant junk food abuse. What's needed is a brand new 'workforce' to come in and clean the rubbish out. The body was simply never designed to cope with the barrage of slow, hard-to-digest food that we chuck down our gullet on a daily basis. I am not saying that it cannot cope with this junk to some degree, because it can. In fact if the body is genuinely hungry it will digest almost anything – but only a *certain amount* of anything. However, if it is starved of life, and at the same time is asked to do more and more work with little or no tools, it will slowly crumble and everything you do will feel equivalent to climbing a mountain.

The human body was specifically designed with fast food in mind, and again I don't mean burgers and KFC. I mean foods that are fast to digest, fast for the body to assimilate (take what it needs for human function and growth) and fast for the body to eliminate. I mean real, genuine fast food – a set of foods that will quickly inject nutrients into every cell in your body, giving it a brand new workforce that is specifically designed to clear out excess fat and waste. A set of foods that contain massive amounts of what our body thrives on – water, which flushes out waste matter and keeps oxygen flowing in the system. And this amazing group of foods also replenishes your enzyme bank account, keeping you slim, and looking and feeling fantastic.

I will give you plenty of examples of true fast foods soon and I will be explaining how you can produce a truly amazing fast food, one that is so powerful that it literally blasts fat from cells, clears the skin and releases bundles of energy. It is what I call *the fastest food in the west* and is the single most powerful physical weapon against fat, ageing and lethargy. But before I do there are a lot of myths to shatter and there is one particular junk food which ranks supreme in the slow-to-be-digested, assimilated and eliminated steaks (pun intended). Yes, I am talking about a junk food which for many years we were told we couldn't live without: a food which many still believe is vital for our well-being and survival, but one which many don't realize can be...

15

A Meaty Problem

Meat – a problem? 'But it's full of iron, protein, vitamins and minerals. It's the bedrock of any decent meal; it's what keeps us strong, healthy and bouncing with energy. What would Christmas or Sunday dinner be without the "bird" or a joint of meat? What about barbecues? What about pork crackling, rib-eye steak and, oh my God, what about bacon sarnies?'

The truth is, if you were to eliminate meat you would probably be a lot healthier, you would certainly have more energy and you could still enjoy social occasions. However, you don't have to stop eating meat altogether in order to be healthy. But there are a few things you may like to know about this apparent 'health' food if your goal is a slim body and bundles of energy.

This subject really does require an open mind. Some people have such deep-rooted beliefs, often installed since early childhood, that they are unwilling to entertain the idea that meat could be a bad thing. To be fair, I was one of them. For a few years I worked in a butcher's shop, my uncle's to be precise, but I was never a butcher (my uncle would be the first to agree with that). As you can imagine I had a pretty strong belief that meat was simply the best thing you could eat. I was constantly surrounded with posters which read 'Protein, vitamins, minerals, iron and two veg', 'Meat To Live', 'Lamb for Lovers' and the like. All this, of course, backed up everything my teachers, family and even my doctor had told me ever since I could communicate. It seems we have all been somewhat hoodwinked for many years about the subject of meat. We have been conditioned to believe that unless you eat meat you will not get enough protein, be lacking in vitamin B_{12} and be weak and feeble. I would like to dispel a few of the myths, especially the ones about meat providing strength and energy. So forget what you have read or been taught for a few minutes and let's use our common sense.

Have you seen the size of an elephant? Pretty big aren't they? Would you say they are strong? Not many Benny! They are not just strong, they are *the* strongest land animal in the world. Have you any idea the amount of meat they eat to maintain the massive strength they have? None, zero, diddly squat – not even a sausage. They don't eat any meat yet are hardly lacking in the strength or energy department now are they? Even our closest living relatives, the great apes, only eat meat in emergencies and once again they are hardly built like Kate Moss. They are three times as heavy and thirty times as strong as the average human and yet their diet consists mainly of nature's fast food – fruit. And bear in mind that their digestive system is still virtually identical to ours. If they do have to eat meat in order to stay alive – they eat it raw (this means it still contains enzymes and these help with digestion, assimilation and disposal). You don't see a group of silverbacks cooking up a tee-bone on the barbie now do you? So now you might be thinking '*raw* – err how disgusting, we would never do that.' Exactly, that's the point. For most of us the thought of eating raw meat is disgusting – we have to cook it in order to try and make it edible. Even before it's cooked many meats have to be 'hung' for many days to try and make them tender in order to make them even remotely palatable for humans. If you tried to hang meat for a week in the wild someone would soon nick it!

So not only is the meat we eat not fresh; it is often very old. Any enzymes that may be left in it we totally destroy by cooking it. Please remember that when you cook anything above 118°F (a temperature that is too low to even register on most cookers) you kill it. We were told for years that we should cook food in order to destroy all of the harmful bacteria and, yes, when you cook some foods, this is what you do. But what else do you think you might be killing at the same time? *All* of the live nutrients. You simply can't destroy one with destroying the other. When I was growing up I had to live with my aunt for a year. She used to start cooking the Sunday dinner at about 9am! By the time the meal was served there was more nutrition left on the kitchen walls and ceiling than was left in the food. I now understand why food smells so good when it's cooking – it's all the goodness coming *out*.

So am I suggesting you eat raw meat? No. In order to make it remotely edible we do have to cook it (though some people do eat steak virtually raw). Am I suggesting you eat no meat at all? Again no, not unless you choose not to. What I will suggest, however, is that you follow a few guidelines. When natural omnivores eat meat, they do not eat it at the same time as other difficult-to-digest foods, and they don't eat it that often. They also do not have an already beaten-up digestive system and they eat tons of high-water-content 'live' foods that are packed with enzymes and energy. All of this enables them to easily and comfortably deal with the small amount of meat they do consume. It follows then that our bodies can easily cope with 'some' meat – provided we have the enzymes to deal with it, and we don't expect our body to cope with it at the same time as a whole load of other difficult-to-digest foods.

THE ULTIMATE SLOW FOOD

In terms of digestion, however, huge clumps of meat really are a problem. Meat is what I describe as the ultimate slow food. It takes a great deal of nerve energy to digest and use the stuff. I have said that in order to shift stored fat and increase energy levels, you have to 'free up' energy in the body and at the same time supply oxygen and nutrients to your cells. The easiest way to do this is to eat and drink the Juice Master's 'fast food' and drastically reduce – though not necessarily eliminate – the slow food (junk). Meat is a junk food not a drug food (although with the amount of chemicals and hormones being pumped into many animals that point is now debatable, so go for organic where you can). Red meat, in particular, takes a great deal of time to digest, it is very slow to leave the stomach, very slow at getting through the intestinal tract and very slow to be eliminated. In fact red meat can be so hard for an already-tired system to fully eliminate that often it never *fully* leaves the body. This is not simply hearsay. When the actor John Wayne died of colon cancer they found 14lb of rotting flesh in his colon. It has been said that the average, regular red meat eater will end up with anything from 2–16lb of decaying flesh in their colon by the time they are 50.

When Ivan Pavlov, the famous 'bell' man, researched how long certain foods took to be digested he discovered that meat stays in the stomach for an average of four hours when it is eaten alone. This time is apparently more than doubled if you add a load of potato and Yorkshire pudding at the same time (more about combining foods in a sec). Now when I first heard that I thought 'so what?' Well it turns out that fruit, for example, only stays in the stomach for about half an hour – that's *fast* food. Fresh juice or smoothies only take about 15 minutes – the Juice Master's *fastest food in the west*. The reason meat is there for so long is because the body has to work hard trying to digest it before it passes it through the intestines. It finds the task difficult because we only have a tenth of the hydrochloric acid that natural carnivores have. Hydrochloric acid is the acid the body uses to break down the toxins in meat. It seems fairly obvious that humans were not meant to deal with meat on a regular basis as we have such a small amount of the acid needed to digest meat properly. At the same time the saliva we produce is alkaline, yet the saliva of *all* carnivores is acid. We also have an incredibly long intestinal tract, while all meat eating animals in the wild have very short intestines. This enables the meat to pass through quickly to avoid putrefaction. Nature designed food for every creature to be as fast as possible. The time it actually takes for meat to pass through the entire gastrointestinal tract just might surprise you – 72 hours! Meat is broken down a lot quicker if it's eaten at the same time as some high-water-content, nutrient-packed salad or vegetables. The nutrients help to digest it and the high water content helps to transport it through the body.

The truth is that meat is so far from what we would naturally eat that we even have to rename the stuff in order to eat it. When I worked at the butcher's shop, if someone came in and asked what I recommended for a barbecue I never said 'How about some pigs' heads that have been crushed, boned and minced with some added water, chemicals, rusk and encased in small tubes of pigs' intestines'. Somehow I don't think I would have sold too many if I had! No, I would say, 'How about some sausages'. Children have no idea what they are eating. Ask the average child where their bacon sandwich came from they will say Sainsbury's or Tesco. Somehow I don't think they would get as much joy if, whilst they were watching the film *Babe*, we broke the hard truth to them.

MYSTERY FOOD

It wouldn't be so bad if we were eating organic whole meats, but often the meat we are eating is not only not organic or whole but it's part of the 'mystery' food group. Chicken burgers, beef burgers, chicken Kiev, chicken nuggets, sausages, hot-dogs etc. are all examples of mystery foods – meaning it's a complete mystery what's really in them. What you think you are getting is often not meat at all but a load of synthetic, man-made, chemically-bound 'foodstuffs' – a small percentage of which might actually be some meat. I mean a hot-dog, what the hell is in it?

And don't be fooled by the many fast food outlets that boast about their burgers being 100 per cent pure beef. By 100 per cent pure beef they mean 100 per cent pure cow. Which includes the colon, the intestines, the liver, the kidneys, the spleen – just about everything in fact.

So my advice is to skip the frozen meat meals like chicken Kiev and stick to organically produced (very hard when out having a meal, I know), *whole* meats. At least that way you know it is chicken, or turkey, or whatever. When it is encased in breadcrumbs or a pig's intestine it becomes a 'mystery food'. Please also note that organic white meats are nowhere near as acidic to the body as red meat and the body has a much easier time dealing with them, so if you want some organic chicken with steamed veg and a water-rich, nutrient-packed salad it will not interfere with your success – in fact it's an extremely healthy meal. The general rule if you are still going to consume meat is nothing from a cow or pig where possible.

CARNIVORES? OMNIVORES? HERBIVORES?

There has been a lot of argument about whether we were designed to eat meat or not. After reading the evidence on both sides, and believe me I've read loads of it, I have once again used the best resource I know to come up with my own conclusion – common sense. All I know is that if I was in the wild and had the choice between picking a banana from a tree next to me or chasing down an animal, I'd choose the banana. It's much easier than catching, killing and cutting up an animal. But if I was hungry and there wasn't any fruit available, and *all* that was left were some animals roaming around, then watch out 'Babe' – I'm coming to get ya! We would eat anything rather than starve and in times of genuine hunger your body can easily cope with meat.

So in terms of whether you *can* eat meat or not the answer is clear – yes we can. In terms of whether we actually need it to live the answer is also very clear – no we don't. The meat industry, along with various government agencies, have managed to convince seemingly everyone that unless we get tons of protein we will die. They have also managed to convince us that meat is the best source of this much-needed protein. Massive advertising campaigns like the 'Meat to Live' one constantly back up this huge myth we've been taught since birth – so let's lay this one to rest once and for all.

WE JUST DON'T NEED THAT MUCH PROTEIN

Think about it. In the first six months of life we literally double in body weight. At no other point in our life does this happen in such a short amount of time (although it can often feel as though it does). We need more protein during the first few years of our life than at any other time. And the reason – the body is growing nails, hair, bones, tissues, etc. It needs a good source of protein for this – namely mother's milk. Here's the thing, mother's milk contains a *maximum* of 2.2 per cent protein. Also, protein is not built from protein anyway – it is built from amino acids. The reason we eat cows is because apparently their protein is very similar to ours – which seems like a very good argument for eating your next door neighbour! And what is all the fear about not getting enough protein anyway? Where did this fear come from? Have you ever met anyone with a protein deficiency? No, me neither. But I have met loads of people suffering the effects of *too much* protein. It is up to you to use your common sense, but if you are in any doubt just ask yourself, where do cows get their protein from?

'Are you telling me I have to eat grass to get my protein?'

No, I'm saying it seems that whatever food was specifically meant for each species has exactly the correct amount of protein – despite what the 'experts' may say. The closest living relative to us is the Bonobo chimpanzee. In fact this species is closer to us genetically than it is to any other chimpanzee. Our digestive systems are virtually identical and our DNA is 98 per cent the same. They eat nothing but fruit and green leafy vegetation, yet they are very strong and powerful. I am not suggesting that we need to do this for a second, so don't panic, I am just pointing out that once again we have been handed a load of clap-trap when it comes to the protein and meat issue.

Let's be very clear – our bodies *were* designed to deal with meat, but not all the time and not at least without the help of nutrient-packed, water-rich live food to help it along. If you have meat once, twice, even three times a week it will cause you no problems whatsoever and you will still easily and comfortably arrive safe in Mauritius – especially if you change your brand to white meat. In fact, if that's all you're having, it will probably be of benefit to you. Equally, not having meat will also cause you no problems whatsoever either. The question of meat comes down to not whether you can, but whether you really want to.

I haven't eaten meat for many years now, but I must stress I am not a vegetarian, and I must say that I was eating meat throughout the time I shed the weight, got slim and replenished my energy bank account. In other words I arrived safe and sound in Mauritius while I was still eating meat. I am also not saying that I will never eat it again, as there may be times in my life where meat may be the *only* half decent option. There might also be times when I'm in a different country and just want to experience a particular dish – when in Rome and all that. The idea is to understand the effect meat can have on your system, and then to be flexible and free to eat it intelligently.

I DON'T EAT MEAT BUT I'M NOT A VEGETARIAN

Now what do I mean by that? Well, although I don't eat meat (except 'When in Rome'), I do eat fish, which apparently makes me a 'pescitarian' (I wonder who came up with that beauty). The body can deal with fish a lot, and I mean a hell of a lot, easier than even white meat. It also contains some essential fats we need, along with the essential amino acids which are the building blocks of protein. Although you can easily get these fats from avocados and nuts, and amino acids from pulses, grains and nuts, I sometimes just like a piece of hot cooked fish on a bed of water-rich, live salad – especially if I'm eating in a restaurant.

Personally I've never understood people who claim they are vegetarian and yet eat fish. Apparently there are even people who claim to be veggie and justify it by saying, 'I don't eat meat apart from chicken and fish'. That's like saying I don't smoke apart from pipes and cigars. Fish is classed as a Juice Master junk food, but it does not take anything like the same amount of time to digest and use as meat. In fact, I am loath to put the word fish and junk in the same sentence, because fish can be extremely beneficial, but for the purposes of my definition it is classed as junk (though it's in a different league from meat and personally I eat it quite often).

Many people think that if they stopped eating meat they would miss the wonderful taste if it, but remember the chapter on 'changing your brand'. You will learn to enjoy the taste of anything you have on a regular basis and most people already like at least some kinds of fish. And anyway, meat has never really tasted that good and has always been a bit dull. Why do you think we add salt, pickle, ketchup and the like? With foods that we are biologically adapted to eat we don't need to add stuff to improve the taste, and we also do not need to rename them. You don't have to rename an apple, a pear or a banana to make it mentally acceptable, and you certainly don't need to add ketchup or pickle to a pineapple to 'improve' the taste. But remember –

You do not have to stop eating meat altogether to be slim and healthy

Far from it, so if you don't want to stop eating meat altogether – DON'T. If you enjoy your turkey or chicken at Christmas then have it. If you want a Sunday roast – enjoy. If you like a nice bit of chicken on the barbie – feel free to tuck in. In fact, if you are ever in the position where you have a choice between a plate full of white pasta and some meat and veg, go with the meat and veg every time (as you will see very soon). Good quality whole meats are not the real enemy here – it's the mystery food 'meats' and drug foods that you've got to look out for. Whole meats are only a problem when we burden our system with *too much* at the cost of everything else. In fact, if you look around there are many vegetarians who are fat and incredibly unhealthy. The main reason for this is that most people who stop eating meat still haven't got it quite right – they simply substitute meat with an even more toxic junk food. Although they call themselves vegetarians they really are more like…

16

'Dairy'-arians

'Dairy what?' Dairyarians. I wouldn't look it up as I made up the word. The point is many people who stop eating meat start eating loads of dairy products which, in terms of weight and health, are a nightmare.

For many years we have all been bombarded with nonsense about this 'apparent' health food. 'Apparent health food?' I hear you holler. Yes, *apparent* health food. The dairy industry has literally been 'milking' us for years. Not only did they manage at one time to make milk compulsory in schools, but even today doctors, dieticians and a host of other 'experts' still insist that milk is good for us and without it our bones and teeth would crumble. I have just one thing to say about most of what we have been taught about milk and dairy products and that is…

Bullshit

Have you seen the teeth of a great ape? Do you know how much milk they drink? None. Do the great apes have bones in their body? I should say so – big, strong and very healthy bones. In fact, come to think of it, not one single adult mammal drinks milk after they are weaned – except of course us. Even a cow doesn't drink milk, which is worth thinking about perhaps – calves do, but cows don't. That is because it is completely unnatural for any mammal to drink milk of any kind after they are weaned. It is even more unnatural (after weaning age) to drink the milk of a completely different species.

If you are thinking that cats and dogs drink milk, bear in mind who controls what they eat. Cats and dogs are now suffering many of the diseases we have and many are now very fat indeed. If humans were meant to have any kind of milk it should of course be from our own mother – not the mother of a calf. But mother's milk either dries up or it becomes very uncomfortable for the mother to continue, hence we, like all mammals, should be weaned off milk at an early age. You can try and get some mother's milk now if you like. But be warned – you'll get arrested!

The milk of a cow is clearly meant for its own kind and I don't care how many people with qualifications coming out of their ears say otherwise. It is meant for a mammal that has a digestive system with *four* stomachs; one which weighs an average of 200lb at birth and 2000lb just two years later. If you want that kind of weight gain then carry on consuming this stuff. But bear in mind why milk and dairy produce causes so many problems for so many humans – it was meant for a completely different species. Often health problems are never put down to the milk such is the power of belief that the milk of a cow is good for a human. For example, I was badly asthmatic for many years and wouldn't go anywhere without my inhalers. I had both the blue and brown versions and was taking puffs on them at least eight times a day. Within just four weeks of eliminating milk products from my diet I no longer had asthma and I haven't had it since. I am not saying that if you have asthma your problem will certainly be solved by avoiding milk, but you can be almost certain it will be drastically improved. Why? Because milk and dairy products are mucus forming. That mucusy, sticky stuff can build up and get stuck to parts of your breathing apparatus. Why does it do this to the inside of a human? Because we shouldn't be drinking it! The mucus build-up is somewhat of an 'action signal'. It is the body's way of saying, 'I am having difficulty dealing with this rubbish, if possible, please don't do it again'. But how on earth are we meant to recognize and act on these signals when we have been told by experts that milk is good for us. Because of this conditioning we often put the many problems that milk causes down to other causes, and continue to drink and eat products made from this glue-like substance.

Because of all the nonsense that has been said about this foodstuff I feel I need to explain in very simple terms some things you really *do* need to know. Milk contains a protein called casein; it also, as you are no doubt aware, contains calcium. The casein and calcium are chemically bound together. In order for the protein to be used efficiently and the calcium to be utilized properly the body requires certain digestive enzymes to split them up. These enzymes are called rennin and lactase. Here's the problem – if you are human and are over the age of three (I should well imagine that includes you) you will no longer have these enzymes (some humans do continue to produce lactase, but it is rare). Do you think there might be a blatantly obvious reason why our bodies stop producing the enzymes that break down milk properly after the age we are meant to be weaned?

LINING YOUR STOMACH WITH GLUE

It's tough enough for the body to deal with human milk after weaning age, but at least this was meant for an animal with one stomach – us. This is why goat's milk is better for humans than cow's milk – they also only have one stomach. But just because it's *better* doesn't mean it's good. Once again this milk was meant for 'kids' *not* the goat and not for us either. Both goat's milk and cow's milk contain a much higher amount of the protein casein than human milk and it's this stuff which is a major problem for our digestive system. In fact, cow's milk contains over 300 times more casein than human milk. 'So what' I hear you say 'isn't casein protein? The more the better surely'. Hardly, casein is one of the strongest wood glues known to mankind. It literally sticks to the walls of the stomach and lining of the intestines. The mad thing is we know this but we just don't think about it. How many times have you heard people say, 'I'm going to have a few beers tonight, but before I do I'm going to line my stomach with milk'? And that really is what's happening – you're lining your stomach and intestines with a glue-like substance. In terms of weight gain it's a nightmare, as any good food you eat cannot be absorbed properly and the bad stuff cannot be passed out. If bad stuff cannot be passed out it will be stored and for so many people the toxic waste matter gets stored in fat cells. Even if you are not overweight, you will slowly become more lethargic and tired. This is because your breathing apparatus becomes full of mucus, your stomach and intestines lined with a glue-like substance and your bloodstream loaded with animal sugars and fats.

I know this subject often causes controversy and I have had many heated debates with people who are unwilling to let go of their deep-rooted beliefs about this subject (Anna). But it really is hard to argue with plain common sense and my common sense clearly tells me that the milk of a cow is meant for a calf – not a human being. The 'action signals' people get after consuming large amounts also confirm this belief.

There is a massive push for milk going on in the UK as I write this book. The slogan we are hearing over and over again from the milk industry is 'Are you made of the white stuff', which seems a tad ironic given that we really are not made of 'the right stuff' to deal with the white stuff. All I know is that since drastically reducing my intake of dairy products I have tons more energy, no excess weight and I can breathe again.

CHEESED OFF

While we're on the subject, let's not forget that milk is used to make numerous different products, from Yorkshire puddings, biscuits, cakes, chocolate and muffins to the most obvious one – cheese.

Now there are certain action signals that tell which foods we should or should not have. One of the many things which tells us what to eat is our sense of smell. Let me ask you a question on the subject of cheese: what does Parmesan smell of? That's right – sick! Many people say old socks, but either way it smells disgusting. To me it smells of sick. Now I don't know about you but when I eat something I like to enjoy both the taste *and* the smell. This just proves you will learn to like the taste of anything you have on a regular basis, even if it stinks. The reason why Parmesan smells so awful is because it's off – the same goes for all soft blue cheeses too. Do you know how blue cheese is made? They get some solidified cow's milk, put holes in it and leave it until *mould* sets in the holes and settles – 'um'. And we eat this because it's apparently good for our health.

We also do it because, if we are really honest, we get caught up with a lot of the pretentious nonsense that surrounds so many foods. Someone eating a Cheddar sandwich, drinking a can of beer, with a fag hanging out of their mouths, is seen as being different to someone with a piece of stilton, biscuits, a glass of white wine and a 'fine' cigar – yet they're consuming the same stuff. In fact the person with the blue cheese is eating added mould. It seems strange that the more something has gone off the more 'sophisticated' it becomes and the more we seem willing to pay for it. Children usually hate blue cheese; Cheddar is about as much as they can stomach (so to speak). We have to 'acquire' a taste for tangy, often very bitter cheese and the only reason we do is to 'fit in' with a certain image.

'But Jason, if I do choose to get rid of meat from my diet and drastically reduce or eliminate dairy products, where will I get my protein and calcium – and what about vitamin B_{12}?'

The above seems like a reasonable question, but only because of the conditioning and misinformation we have been subjected to since birth. An elephant wouldn't worry about where it's getting its protein or vitamin B_{12} and it certainly doesn't give a hoot about calcium. The irony is that people who eat animal products have a much *higher* incidence of B_{12} deficiency problems. I haven't eaten meat in years, I was also a vegan for a couple of years, but I am hardly wasting away. I really don't care about vitamin B_{12} and neither should you. Once again it falls in the ever-increasing category of – WE DON'T NEED TO KNOW.

It always seems very odd to me that people start to get concerned about whether they are getting enough vitamins, minerals, protein and calcium *after* they change their diet. When they are eating nothing but McDonalds, ice cream, processed and totally de-natured foods, they don't seem that worried. But the minute you talk about having fresh fruit, veg and freshly extracted juice, they start to worry: why? Because the meat and dairy industries have perpetuated fears for many years that are totally unfounded – like the one about not getting enough calcium. I know I have repeatedly said that we really do not need to concern ourselves with the likes of calcium, but in order to put your unfounded fears to rest there are a few things you *should* know.

The main use of calcium is to help neutralize acid in the body. This means that every time you put something acid forming in your body you rob your bank account of calcium. Our bank balance is mainly stored in our bones and teeth. Luckily we have quite a hefty bank account but, once again, if you keep withdrawing without making deposits you will go bankrupt. And when the body files for calcium bankruptcy the consequence is brittle bones and loss of teeth. In fact osteoporosis (brittle bone disease) is now a common condition – and it's common because of what we are putting into our bodies. However, if what they say about dairy products and calcium is true, this should not be happening. Our intake of dairy products has gone *up* drastically over the past thirty years, yet so has the rate of osteoporosis.

The fact is most people have got it back to front. They are so busy worrying about where they are going to get more calcium from that they don't think about what's depleting their current store. As usual we are so busy treating the symptom we don't look for the cause. Every time you drink coffee, cola or alcohol, smoke a cigarette, or eat a fast-food burger your body has to use its calcium stores to help neutralize the acid effect they have on the body. The question is not where do I get my calcium, but rather how can I prevent the scavengers coming in and taking it all? And bear in mind that cow's milk has an acid effect in the human body.

Milk products are used in massive quantities by many of the fast food giants. The most obvious place they use it is in milk shakes, but it is also found in their pastries, biscuits, doughnuts, chocolate sauces, ice creams and the slices of plastic-looking worryingly yellow cheese you find in your cheeseburger. And, if we can get it up the straw, we try and wash this down with a thick, glue-like milkshake.

Having said all of this, dairy produce, just like meat, is classed as a junk food and not a drug food (although again many versions do contain chemicals, rendering them drug foods). This means that you do not have to eliminate it completely in order to have excellent health and bundles of energy. Personally, although I went two years without eating any dairy products whatsoever, I do now eat cheese every so often and if I ever do have a jacket potato I will certainly add some butter. Clearly I choose a good organic source of dairy, where possible, but yes, at times I'll even have cheese *with* the butter on a jacket – so shoot me! Remember, it's what you do *most* of the time that determimnes your health; the body will easily cope with a *bit* of dairy and the whole point of this book is the freedom of *genuine* food choice. But please bear in mind that just as fish is classed as the easiest Juice Master junk food for your body to gain something from, dairy produce is the worst and due to the often high levels of lactose (milk sugar) is a borderline drug food. However, if you want *some* cheese on your salad, feel free, the body will cope. Always remember that the body can easily deal with a *certain amount* of just about anything, especially when it is in an excellent state of health. But please also bear in mind that for most people I see – and the same will go for most people reading this book – their body, or 'industry' as I call it, is already running very low on energy. It has also lost valuable staff over the years, has an already weak digestive tract and the last thing it needs is to be covered in glue whilst trying to eliminate stored poisons. So while you're on your flight to Mauritius I'd skip the cow glue as much as possible.

The Juice Master programme is one you can use every day for life and the key is flexibility and common sense. Have meat if you want it and the 'odd' bit of dairy produce too and don't have a nervous breakdown over it. Once you have live nutrients flowing through every cell in your body (provided, of course, by the power of juice and fresh whole foods), you can rest assured it will easily cope with the odd piece of white meat or dairy produce. It's only when the body is flooded with this stuff and is lacking in vital nutrients that the problems occur. The body was designed to eat anything in an emergency, but it just wasn't designed to be in a permanent state of red alert.

I realize there may be many vegetarians reading this book who are now perhaps realizing they are in fact more like dairyarians and as such are doing their health and energy levels no favours at all. I know many vegetarians who are in fact *dairyarians*, but these people went veggie for two reasons – health and animal welfare. The problem is they fall flat on both counts. If it's for health then they are certainly not better off substituting milk products for meat products. Given the choice between a veggie cheese-ridden lasagne and some chicken and steamed veg – go for the meat every time! And as for animal welfare (which I realize is a totally different subject), they certainly haven't done anything to help the cause as dairy herds go through much worse torture than those reared for slaughter only.

Now that you are aware of the pitfalls of being a dairyarian you're probably thinking of a substitute food. If you are, please be careful not to make the next big mistake – that of turning into a 'starcharian'. This is a person who, you guessed it, eats tons of bread, rice, potatoes, corn and pasta at the cost of most other things. In terms of getting slim, healthy and tapping into a level of energy you haven't felt in years, you are better off eating some meat, a *little* dairy produce every now and then and saying…

17

Pasta la
Vista Baby

'Are you a couple of penne tubes short of a full dish? Say goodbye to my pasta, is that what you are suggesting? Have you gone mad Jason? Pasta is full of fibre and essential carbohydrates, and it's quick and easy. The Italians thrive on it and it tastes wonderful. So why do we need to say goodbye to pasta?'

Well actually you don't need to say goodbye to pasta at all, you just need to 'change your brand' to the whole-food varieties – and the same goes for bread and rice. The mistake people tend to make when they cut down on meat and dairy produce, is to drastically increase their intake of white refined carbs, which, as you now realize, in terms of health, energy, addiction and weight gain, are a nightmare. I cannot repeat enough how harmful – both in terms of mental addiction and physical abuse – these white refined trashy foods are. When you eat these 'empty' foods you will feel empty and, along with your blood sugar levels shooting sky high then crashing, you will get massive energy slumps throughout the day. This in turn causes a need for pick-me-ups (more drug foods and drinks) like coffee or more refined white sugar products. These cause short, tiny *false* boosts in the blood, which will again cause the body to slump even further. When it does, the need for a pick-me-up will be even greater and, slowly but surely, the nightmare gets worse and worse and the loop continues.

Always keep it clear in your mind that it is not just white refined sugar that causes massive problems, it's *any* white refined carbohydrate. They are the insulin-producing, fat-causing, energy-zapping, stomach-bloating, paste-forming, empty drug-like foods that help to keep people rooted in the food trap. If you want true freedom from the trap and a slim, energy-driven body, then you must say –

Good riddance to white rubbish

This does not mean you cannot have complex carbohydrates and still be healthy, it just means the answer is to switch to the 'whole' varieties of these foods. That way you can still have pasta, rice and bread but in a form that will not do you as much harm. 'Do you mean even these are not good?'. Yes, even with the whole varieties, too much and your sugar levels can creep up causing insulin to be produced and lethargy to set in. Also, some of the wholemeal breads you find in mass quantity at supermarkets contain hydrogenated vegetable oils, sugar (yes sugar), salt, plus various other ingredients not really conducive with human consumption. They are also, like pasta, loaded with wheat. Despite wheat being given a 'good health' image it's yet another food which isn't all it's cracked up to be. Many people are now what's called 'wheat intolerant' and 'wheat free' foods are rapidly finding their way onto many supermarket shelves. One of the biggest problems with wheat, especially for those looking to drop the excess pounds, is water retention. To be fair you hardly need to be a scientist to have already worked this out. Have you ever noticed how your stomach sticks out after eating a load of pasta or bread? That's primarily the wheat! You don't get this so much when you eat rice do you? This is why I'm a big fan of wholegrain rice and less of a fan of wholemeal bread and pasta. Again, don't get me wrong, these wholemeal versions are in a completely different league to their white trashy cousins and I'm *not* saying they're bad foods, I'm just saying if you want that elusive flat stomach, when you *do* eat them – GO EASY ON THE WHEAT!

Wholemeal and whole-grain versions satisfy your hunger for longer as their energy is released steadily, unlike the 'up and crash' cycle you get with the 'refined' white versions. The body also requires fibre, and *whole-grain* rice and good quality bread can be the next best thing to fruit and veg for helping to 'sweep' the intestines. The fibre also helps to slow the rate at which the complex carbs are converted to glucose. Plus, of course, this way of eating is for the rest of your life, so it's important to still have *some* complex carbs. The trick is to have a full understanding of the foods available to us and know exactly which brands to have, as well as how much our bodies can 'get away with' and still stay slim and have optimum health.

WATCH OUT FOR THE YEAST 'PARASITES'

Most of the breads we buy also contain a lot of yeast and many people consume far too much due to their addiction to white carbs – another excellent reason for changing brands. Over consumption can eventually cause an overgrowth of yeast in the gut (otherwise known as candida albicans), which in turn causes yet more cravings. Imagine a colony of yeast parasites living in the body. The more you feed them, the more they breed. The more they breed, the more yeast they crave to try and satisfy their insatiable appetite. Have you ever noticed that green hairy mould you get on old bread? Well now imagine an overgrowth of virtually the same mould inside your body with living parasites buried within. That is candida albicans – lovely. All white refined sugar products help to feed the little blighters, as does the sugar found in milk.

Please understand again that a certain amount of both yeast and wheat is fine and some people reading this book will not have these 'parasites'. But at the same time there will be many people who do and those who do often suffer from bloating and fatigue directly after eating white refined pasta, bread and the like. If you have an unusual craving for bread and/or pasta you can be almost certain it's not *you* who wants it, it's the yeast, wheat and sugar parasites within. The answer is to realize it's not a genuine hunger and starve the little blighters to death. It is also worth pointing out that white refined flour when mixed with water creates a paste that would be worthy of any roll of wallpaper! Your body is over 70 per cent water and when you ingest flour it becomes like thick paste in your bloodstream, often sticking to the walls of your arteries. Potato crisps also have this effect.

CARBO-*DE*-HYDRATE

Carbohydrates are designed to supply energy, vitamins, minerals, essential fats, amino acids (building blocks for protein) fibre *and* water. With that in mind it seems rather odd that things like flour and wheat are described are 'hydrates'. Carbohydrate actually comes from the fact that carbs such as fruits and veg are very high in water, which is essential for the body. Even a banana is made up of over 84 per cent water. Remember, carbohydrates are designed to supply energy *and* water. However, the complex carbs we eat, even of the whole-grain kind, are lacking in the water. This is why I often refer to them as just carbs, as the hydrate part is not strictly appropriate. This is why when I do have carbs I make sure the hydrate part comes from water-rich foods and vegetable juices.

The bread I eat now tends to be wholemeal pitta bread, which I stuff with loads of water-rich, nutrient-packed fast foods – creamy avocados, fresh tomatoes, alfalfa sprouts, cucumber, lemon juice etc. Wholemeal pittas contain very little yeast and not massive amounts of wheat either and so help to starve yeast parasites, but at the same time allow you to eat 'normally'. I also at times have pumpernickel, rye, stone-ground, buckwheat and *whole*meal breads. The key word is 'whole'. White refined is 'empty' food – anything that was ever good about the grain has been totally removed, rendering it dead and, as you by now should realize, dangerous! So when buying any grains you need to look for the closest to the original *whole* versions as possible – *whole* oats, *whole*meal bread, *whole*-grain brown rice, whole, whole, whole! Plus, unlike the white trashy dangerous variety, *whole* complex carbs can actually help to regulate insulin, stabilize blood-sugar levels and keep things moving – if you know what I mean! They also contain some valuable nutrients which can be *easily* absorbed by the body. So as you can see I'm not suggesting for one second you say goodbye to pasta, bread, rice and oats – just *change your brand*.

As you might be aware it's tricky trying to get wholemeal breads and whole-grain pasta in restaurants. The answer is to choose something else from the menu, such as a chicken or fish dish with some steamed veg, a large salad or even some mashed potato. You can, of course, have the odd bit of white pasta in an emergency. I cannot repeat enough that the body was designed to deal with a certain amount of anything when it is genuinely hungry, but also remember that when it comes to drug-like foods, the mind wasn't designed to cope. White refined sugars, breads, rice and pasta create empty feelings and unless recognized for what they are can cause a person to slip back into the food trap. I tend to stay pretty clear of white refined carbs and even in an Italian restaurant I order a big salad or a fish dish. The only time I eat it is when it really is the *only* thing available, for instance when I'm at someone's house for a meal or at a set menu dinner. Other than that I stay well clear as it's one of the biggest causes of obesity, lethargy and diabetes in the world. Please also be aware that yeast 'parasites' simply love refined carbs and will continue to thrive if this stuff is readily available.

So, once again, the question is not whether you *can* have white refined pasta, bread and rice – after all you are an adult and you can do what you want – but whether you really *want* to. Personally I have no desire to flood my body with a fat-producing, energy-stealing, empty non food – especially when there are millions of high-fibre, nutrient-packed, energy-releasing foods on offer. Just because I don't eat drug-like food doesn't mean I am being restricted or deprived, in fact it's now the opposite – I am finally free of having to try and control a lot of the time and my body is no longer in a permanent state of feeling deprived.

As you can now see, meat, dairy produce and refined carbs all create their own challenges for the body to overcome. Dairy produce, in my opinion, is the worst because of its glue-like effect and the fact that it prevents the good stuff you do eat from being absorbed and the bad stuff from being passed out. This is very closely followed by paste-like, insulin-producing white refined flour, which is then followed closely by red meat. A little way behind these are white meat and whole-grain complex carbs, with fish being the best by far of this bad bunch. I must repeatedly say that I'm loath to put the words *bad*, whole-grain carbs, white lean meats and fish in the same sentence. These foods *can* indeed be *extremely beneficial* as long as they are either eaten by themselves or, better still, with some high-water-content, nutrient-packed JM fast food. Always remember –

The human body was specifically designed to deal with a certain amount of 'junk' without getting diseased

So there is no need to stop having dinner parties, eating carbs, fish or even lean white meat and there is no need to start eating nothing but grass! Don't panic – you will see clearly by the end of this book that you will be free to eat and drink whatever you wish, whenever you wish – this is all about your total freedom from the food trap.

One of the main reasons why many people are lacking in energy and remain fat is because when they do eat these slow, clogging foods, they don't eat them one by one or with any high- water-content JM fast food. The big mistake is that they pile them all in at exactly the same time, course after course, seemingly without worry or care as to what happens *after* they swallow it all. As you now know, each one of these foods affects the body to a greater or lesser degree when eaten *alone*, but put them all together and BOOM! – you've just concocted a very...

18

Lethal Combination

What do Dr William Hay and Ivan Pavlov have in common? They are both scientists who have carried out in-depth studies into the time it takes certain foods and combinations of foods to be digested by the body. In fact, if you are one of these people who have been on the diet roller coaster for years you have by now probably done your own scientific studies into this subject. Whether you have or not, please pay attention to this chapter as you will learn everything you need to know about the effects of shoving all kinds of junk into the body at the same time.

I have already mentioned in 'A Meaty Problem' that our friend Mr Pavlov found that it takes four hours for meat to leave the stomach and a further 20 hours for it to get through the intestinal tract. What I touched on, but have waited until now to expand on, was that the minute you add other concentrated foods (any food which is not fruit, veg or nuts) into the stomach at the *same* time, the overall length of time it takes the body to digest it can more than double. In terms of freeing up energy for weight loss and health this can be a disaster. Here's why.

When you eat a concentrated protein (meat, milk, cheese, fish, eggs, etc.) your body produces *acid*-based digestive juices to help break it down. However, when you put a concentrated starch food (potato, bread, pasta, rice, corn, cereal, oats, rye, etc.) into the body it produces *alkaline*-based digestive juices. 'So what' say you, 'it's all sounding a bit blah, blah, blahish'. Well it's actually worth knowing this bit of blah, blah, blah. Do you remember chemistry lessons at school? Remember what happens when you mix acid and alkaline substances together? They *neutralize* each other – i.e. they cancel each other out. Now because the human body is so efficient, and because the two juices are produced in different parts of the digestive tract, the acid and alkaline juices don't *completely* cancel each other out in this situation (although there are still many 'expert' combining teachers who are convinced they do!). However, there is no question that the body has to work a hell of a lot harder to try and break down *two* concentrated foods at the same time, especially when each require their own specific digestive juice. In fact, the job is made so much harder that the time it takes the stomach alone to deal with this heavy workload will be more than doubled.

Ivan Pavlov recorded that if foods that require different digestive juices are eaten at the same time, it can take anywhere from 8–14 hours for those foods to leave the stomach. To put this in perspective, food should never be in the stomach for longer than 3–4 hours. If it remains there for longer because it is part of a badly combined meal, then putrefaction and fermentation occurs. Meat putrefies and starches like potatoes ferment. Now throw in a cow glue; a highly sugared, theobromine-laced dessert (more carbs and protein); a few alcoholic drinks (carbs plus all kinds of other things) and a couple of cups of coffee – whilst your body is still dealing with meat and potatoes – and you've just put yourself into a slow food coma. Or in our language, we've just nodded off after our Sunday lunch or Christmas dinner.

The other person I mentioned who studied what is now known as 'food combining' is Dr William Hay. As any self-respecting dieter will know, he created the famous Hay Diet. For those who have not only heard of it, but have tried it, please let me put your mind at rest by saying…

This is not a food combining diet

In fact, The Juice Master Programme is not any kind of diet – I'm only mentioning what happens when certain foods hit the stomach to give you an added physical tool to aid in your journey to the land of the slim and healthy.

The Hay Diet was the first in a long line of diets based on the principle that proteins are fine when eaten alone, as are carbs – but never the twain shall meet. In fact this is the whole philosophy behind Slimming World. The difference is they don't just have separate protein and carb meals, they have completely separate days. They have what is known as a Red day and a Green day. Red days are when you can eat your proteins and Green days are for carbs. The theory is obviously based on the findings of Hay and Pavlov, and, because the body is only dealing with one concentrated food at a time, it works – well to a degree anyway. I say to a degree because rarely does *just* separating your carbs and proteins result in the long-term success people are looking for. The main reason is because many people who embark on say the Hay Diet, or are members of a diet club which teaches the same principles, usually still have a diet *mentality* and are often still struggling with other foods and not feeding their body what it needs to get healthy. Usually the only change they make is not mixing proteins and carbs.

The difference for you is that by the time you finish this book you won't have a diet mentality, which means you can easily use food combining as a great physical weapon against fat and ill health whenever *you* choose to. That means when *you* want to and where it fits into *your* life, not constantly so that it dominates your life and you become obsessive about it. In fact, when fully understood and used properly, this combining thing makes an amazing difference to how you feel and really helps to free up valuable nerve energy for weight loss. The difference can be a whooping 5–9 hours of extra energy if you combine sensibly, which is why on the *physical* side of things it's a great tool to have. But in order for it to be an effective tool and one you can use in everyday life in order to have *life-long* success, you need to know the full facts. And once again there are a few myths that need exploding about this combining stuff.

CHINESE WHISPER

If you whisper a truth to someone and ask them to pass the information on, by the time it reaches just the tenth person the facts will have already changed. Exactly the same thing has happened with this combining thing. Very few people have read the original works of Hay or Pavlov. No, what most people have read or heard are simply the headlines and not the full story. Anybody who knows anything about combining tends to believe and purport that you should *never* mix proteins and carbs together no matter what. These are what I call the 'headliners' – people who become so extremely obsessive about not mixing proteins and carbs together that they appear to have convinced themselves they will internally combust if they have a cheese sandwich! I'm not kidding either – I know because on one of my many diets I used to be one of them.

What you need is the full food combining story and not just the headlines. That way you can, as I do now, feel totally relaxed about it and use it to your advantage whenever you wish.

TURNS OUT THE 'WONG WAY' IS THE RIGHT WAY

Once again common sense needs to come into play here. If protein and carbs should *never* be mixed no matter what, why do people in the East – who 'badly combine' all the time – tend to be much healthier and much slimmer than their Western counterparts. (Sadly, things are now changing on this front thanks to the drug food giants moving in.) Also, if the *never* mix proteins and carbs rule is correct then it means that nature herself has got it wrong. After all, she combines proteins and carbs in most of her foods. So how can this be if our friends Hay and Pavlov were correct?

The answer is in the *ratio* of carbs and proteins. In nature, although some proteins will also have carbs, the carbohydrate content will always be low. And in the East they apply the same principles as nature herself when it comes to combining protein and carbs – one or the other always dominates in their dishes. They tend to have lots of rice, plenty of veg and *little* strips of pork, chicken, duck or fish.

Our problem is the result of eating *equal* amounts of protein and carbs at the same time – usually huge clumps of meat and loads of potatoes. And when we do, the undisputed fact is that, yes, it will take double the time to leave the stomach than if they were eaten separately or in the *correct ratio*. The correct ratio means that if you want a *couple* of potatoes with your fish and salad, fine. If you are having a water-rich chicken salad and you want a few chips on the side – have them (yes chips!). The key is not to waste too much energy on digestion. There is a vital reason for this –

It takes energy to lose weight and gain health

I cannot repeat this point enough and this is why one of the biggest changes you need to make is from slow food to fast.

I could spend the next 50 pages on this combining thing, but it would all get a bit blah, blah blahish (if it hasn't already) and I don't want to prattle on unnecessarily. The fact is if you have understood the above, then you now know enough to use combining as a helpful tool to get you to the land of the slim and healthy. The only other things you need to know are a few rules regarding fruit. To prevent us getting distracted now, I have supplied a simple breakdown of all the JM's combining tools at the back for easy reference *after* you have finished the book.

As I have said, the main problem is that many people who follow the Hay and Pavlov school of thought often let this combining stuff rule their entire life. In other words they're not free to eat, which is the whole point of this book. And, as I've said, it's often the only change they make. So initially they will have some weight loss as the body has more energy, but it still won't be enough without a full understanding of the food trap – they will still never feel free or be free. And it's no good simply separating your carbs and proteins if you are still consuming tons of drug foods and drinks and at the same time are still not getting enough vital nutrients. What's the point of a 'Green day' if all you're consuming is tons of white pasta, biscuits, refined sugar and bread. They might all take the same amount of time in the stomach, so therefore are 'correctly combined', but so what! People who have

Green days like this (which ironically can contain no green at all) are not going to achieve the kind of success they're looking for, especially if the pasta and bread are made from white refined trash. And whilst I'm back on that subject please be aware that the drug food industry has no scruples and will deliberately try to delude you into thinking you are eating healthily when you're not. One of the biggest tricks is to literally dye white refined bread with caramel to make it brown. I want to make it clear –

'Brown' bread is just white bread that has been dyed, 'brown' bread is not wholemeal bread – 'brown' bread is a con

And this isn't the only con. Don't be fooled by things like 'brown' sugar either, it's simply white refined sugar that has been dyed – usually with caramel. They just dye it brown to make us think we are getting something healthy. This kind of almost subconscious false advertising really gets on my goat. If you look around they do this type of thing with so many different foods. By adding certain colours to packaging or selective 'buzz' words they attempt, often very successfully, to make us believe that what we are buying is a very healthy food. How they are still allowed to so blatantly mislead the public is a mystery. Before you can free yourself completely from the food trap and change your eating habits for life all of the trickery must be dispelled entirely. So before I get on to explaining how to get into the right frame of mind and exactly how to implement and actively make the change, there are a few more things you should be aware of. The price of not knowing is certain members of the food industry controlling the way we think and raising their glasses as they continue to wish us all a very…

19

Con-appetite

Mainstream advertising on TV and radio and product placement in films conning us into believing certain drug-like foods will change our emotions for the better is bad enough. But perhaps even more sinister is the blatant, subconscious advertising that goes on in the packaging of certain foods. I am talking here about certain buzzwords and colours they use that act like an instant 'bell' to make us believe we are buying something that is good for us. And the reason why we think that foods that are actually rubbish are good for us is not because we are stupid, but because they manage to twist things in such a way that our first impression of the food is 'healthy'. You never get a second chance to make a first impression, as they say, and the manufacturers and advertisers know this.

Some of the biggest buzzwords are GM free, natural and organic. The minute we see these words we believe the product is healthy. But so often it's totally meaningless. Let's look at 'GM free' for a second. GM stands for genetically modified. Many people in the UK became very wary of GM foods in the late '90s because of the massive amount of bad press they were receiving – Prince Charles famously voiced his concerns about them and they were widely referred to as 'Frankenstein' foods. This led to many food manufactures and outlets doing their utmost to inform us that their foods were GM free. This unfortunately gave the very false impression that if something was GM free, it was good for you. Everyone was so busy worrying about GM that they seemed oblivious to the fact that they were still eating foods that were far from healthy.

One of the major UK newspapers even ran a full colour article giving list after list of GM-free foods. They also had a colour scheme to make it easier to see which foods were GM free, which ones contained only a little GM and which contained a lot. The colours they used also helped to confuse people about what is healthy or not. One of the main colours used by so many food manufacturers to fool us into believing we are buying a good food is green. Green is now linked in our minds with health; so much so that all they have to do is add a bit of green to packaging and we become instantly fooled.

In this article on GM foods the colour they used to indicate foods and food outlets that were totally GM free was none other than our natural friend – green. Red was used for places or foods that used a lot of GM and amber for a bit here and there. What seemed a touch mind-blowing to me was that 'restaurants' like McDonalds and KFC were listed in the green column! This indicated that they were totally GM free, but quite frankly – so what, does it really matter? All this means is that the drug-like foods they sell were not genetically modified, but they have still been totally modified from their original state. The sugar started life as part of natural sugar cane; is the stripped, refined version not simply a *modified* version that will cause massive problems to the body? The milkshake certainly didn't start life looking like that and if you think about it I don't think there is one single thing in it that is in its natural state. So as far as I'm concerned I don't care if they're GM free – they are not white refined sugar *free*; refined bread *free*; dairy *free*; meat *free*; high-blood-pressure producing, water-retentive salt *free*; or mystery-food *free*. The fact that they are GM *free* is completely irrelevant to whether they are healthy or not – so don't be fooled. Also bear in mind that EU rules say a product can have 1 per cent GM ingredients without having to declare it anyway.

IT'S ALL NATURAL – BUT THEN SO ARE YOUR CAR TYRES

Another word which has been used for many years to fool us into believing we are eating a good, nutritious, healthy food is 'natural': 'It's all *natural*' or 'Made with only the finest *natural* ingredients' etc. etc. Let's lay this bogie to rest once and for all. If it ultimately came from this planet they are allowed to print 'all natural' on the label if they want to. This seems okay on first hearing but if we really think about the statement it means *anything* that has ever been made must have ultimately come from this planet. Which means that your car tyres, the chair you are sitting on and your clothes are *all natural* – but it doesn't mean they would be good to eat, even if you painted the chair green! My definition of a 'natural' food is any food that is meant for human consumption and still contains *live* nutrients, other than that it's either a drug or junk food – no matter what the label says. Most of the time you can be certain of one thing, most of the labels should be simplified by stating the following:

Nutritional Information – it's all bollocks

That would save us all a lot of time and confusion methinks. Again this doesn't mean you have to live on nothing but live raw foods 24 hours a day to have a slim, energy-driven body. To be honest if you did have to, I would still be fat and lethargic as I still love hot, cooked food on a cold winter's night and love going out for dinner. No, it just means you need a certain amount of live nutrients replenishing your energy bank account in order to *easily* deal with any cooked or processed food you *do* eat. The Juice Master's mental and physical recipe will show you how to easily get the ratio right. But for now I just want you to be very aware of their con tricks.

I have people write down what they ate in the 24 hour period before attending my health seminar. I then ask them what percentage of the food they ate they considered to be natural food. There are many who believe their percentage is 40–50 per cent, when actually it's zero. This is because they are either including meat, dairy, or packaged stuff which was either green in colour or had the word natural, GM free or organic on it.

'Organic' is the biggest buzzword of the moment and it seems anyone who is anyone is now jumping on the bandwagon. They seem to know that the minute we see the word 'organic' printed on virtually any food, our brain immediately thinks it's healthy.

IT'S ORGANIC, SO IT MUST BE GOOD

Yes the organic bandwagon is running at full speed and is being fuelled yet again by a lot of misleading labels and blah, blah, blah talk. So let's cut the crap and spill the organic beans on the way this word often misleads.

Just because a food has the word 'organic' printed on it, IT DOESN'T MEAN IT'S GOOD FOR YOU. Next time you go to your local supermarket just have a look at the amount of drug-like foods with the word 'organic' plastered all over them. You can now even get organic chocolate. Oh so it must be good. There are also organic cakes, organic biscuits, organic crisps, organic tinned sauces, and even organic white refined sugar, bread, rice and pasta.

Can you see how if the words organic and chocolate are used in the same sentence your brain can be deluded into thinking organic chocolate is actually healthy chocolate? And the same goes for virtually any food – if it happens to be made from ingredients which don't contain artificial pesticides, then the word organic can be plastered all over it. But again it doesn't mean it's good, healthy food. It makes no difference if the sugar cane grew without the need for artificial pesticides, it has still been refined and as such is a drug food which causes many problems.

An organically-grown orange is obviously better than an orange which has been grown with artificial pesticides, but if you then take that orange, cook it, add tons of white refined flour and sugar to it then bond it altogether with some glue-like cow's milk it becomes completely irrelevant that the orange *started* its life 'organic'. The process has stripped away anything that was ever good or 'organic'. The orange is now well and truly dead. So if you are going to buy processed, sugar-ridden rubbish, save your money and forget the word 'organic'. Even the 'organic carrot juice' you see in many stores is not worth buying. It may not contain drug-like substances such as sugar, but in order for it to have shelf life they *must* have pasteurized it in some way and as such destroyed *all* the enzymes. The only time organic carrot juice means anything is when you buy one freshly made in front of you at a juice bar.

The words organic or GM free are only significant when we are talking about *fresh* fruit, vegetables, meat, dairy products, wholemeal breads and fish. Although there are many arguments at the moment as to whether organic foods really are better for you or not, I would always recommend organic fresh produce over the rest. Common sense once again tells me that a fresh food that contains added man-made chemicals is bound to be nutritionally inferior to one that doesn't. However, this does not mean that 'normal' fruit and veg are not worth buying if they are not organic – far from it. Please always bear in mind that even with some of the artificial pesticides, fresh fruit and veg are still in a completely different league to drug and junk foods and will always supply the body with plenty of water, nutrients and the *natural* sugars it needs. So if you cannot afford organic produce or it's unavailable – don't worry. This is also where juicing can help as most of the pesticides end up in the 'pulp' (the bit left behind) and not in the juice.

As fish, meat and dairy produce (including eggs) are classed as JM junk foods and not drug foods, most people who have success with this way of thinking *do* continue to eat some foods from these groups. In most cases they have fish a few times a week, meat every now and then and dairy produce as little as possible. With these foods I strongly recommend you buy organic where possible. As I've said before, just because it has the word organic on it doesn't make it good (dairy products in particular will never be good, organic or not) but the organic versions of these foods are often much 'better than' the water-filled, hormone-pumped, steroid-injected, antibiotic-riddled varieties that have been found on many a supermarket shelf over the years.

A wild chicken, for example, would take an average of 7–8 months to grow to its full size, while a commercially-raised chicken can take as little as 7–8 weeks to grow to the same size. How do they make them grow so fast? By pumping them full of steroids and hormones of course. Add to this the antibiotics they are given to prevent the rampant spread of disease common in battery hens and you have a pretty hefty chemical cocktail. And let's not forget BSE or Mad Cow Disease, which was passed on to many humans, particularly in the UK. Okay, so we may be BSE free now but do you really want to be ingesting all those other nasties?

There are several other very misleading statements printed on packets which, despite being totally meaningless, do have an effect on the way we see them. One is –

'Contains real fruit'

Yes we've all seen them, labels on totally rubbish foods giving the already-deceived public the impression that because it contains 'real fruit' it must be good for them. Everyone knows that fruit is without question nature's finest food. It is the most nutritious, the sweetest and the most visually stimulating food on the planet. And that is why the manufacturers and advertisers use it to try and fool us all. By linking whatever totally de-natured product they are trying to sell to the amazing health-giving properties of fresh fruit they persuade us that their product will provide these benefits. I think nature should sue for plagiarism!

What many people do not realize is that once you expose fruit to oxygen it begins to oxidize – or go off. The live nutrients begin to die the minute they are exposed to air. You will have seen this yourself when you have taken a bite of an apple and witnessed how quickly it turns brown – this is the fruit dying. Once dead it is about as much use to the body as the latest state of the art wide-screen TV would be to Stevie Wonder. So whenever you see a tin full of something which contains 'real' fruit – you are guaranteed that the fruit is now dead, destroyed, spent, a total goner. Not only have the life-giving properties of the fruit been totally destroyed, but in order to preserve it you can be sure they have added something which has now turned a perfectly natural food into either a drug or junk food.

The makers of breakfast cereals are perhaps the biggest culprits of this. Many adverts show beautiful colourful images of fruits falling from the sky into a bowl of cereal. They then add a catchy slogan, something like 'as part of a healthy diet' plus the inevitable and misleading, 'May help to keep your heart healthy'. Notice the word MAY. 'May' doesn't mean anything. Nor does 'could', 'possibly', or any of the other rubbish they come out with. I *may* also win the lottery, well I *could* do if I *possibly* had the numbers.

Then you have the drug food pushers whose primary aim is to lure children into buying their particular brand. These people have the front to give the impression to children that things like Starburst and other sweets are in some way good because they show pictures of bright and colourful fruits on their adverts. I want to make this point very clear, unless the fruit is fresh, ripe and whole or the juice freshly extracted, the life-giving properties of the fruit are now gone.

There are many other totally misleading labels such as –

'No artificial colours or flavourings'

Again this gives the impression it's good, but we shouldn't be adding artificial colours in the first place. Not only that but the claim is meaningless as it is often put on products which don't have them anyway, such as pasta or tinned fish. And when they do add colour or flavour to foods they once again try to fool us they are healthy by stating they are 'natural colours' or '*natural* flavourings'. And whilst I'm on the subject, you need to be aware that flavourings and colourings are huge, and I do mean, huge business. The 'flavourists' (yes that's their official title) can make anything taste and smell like anything. That's why so many synthetic lumps of greasy vegetable spreads taste and smell of real butter. Do you know what actually distinguishes a natural flavouring from an artificial one? Well believe it or not the only difference is that a 'natural' flavour is a flavour that's been concocted using an out-of-date technology. What that means is natural and artificial flavours sometimes contain exactly the same chemicals, they're just produced through different methods.

The biggest con of them all though has got to be the 'fat free' and 'low fat' gang. Even Mars brought out an apparently 'healthier' chocolate bar – Mars Flyte low fat chocolate bar. Their slogan: 'Pleasure without the guilt – take flight'. Now I am not into calories and they do fall into the 'we don't need to know category', but in terms of the con it is worth knowing that a Cadbury's Flake has 180 calories and yet the no-guilt Flyte has 196. And when it comes to reducing fat, remember that extra sugar is often added instead – so we're back at the old problem of excess sugar being converted into fat anyway. Peta Cottee of the National Food Alliance sums it up when she states, 'There is no legal definition of what low fat means and shoppers are lulled into a false sense of security when they see these descriptions on labels... Phrases like fat-free are highlighted without it being revealed how much extra sugar may be added to their product'.

'LIGHT' – ON THE TRUTH

Then you have words such as 'light' written all over food that is laced with white refined sugar – the very substance which helps to make people fat and ill! They have pulled the same stroke with cigarettes too. The word 'light' is used on cigarette packets to give the impression that they are healthier, but once again it's all bullshit. The most annoying and unforgiving part about companies shoving words like 'light' or 'fat free' on certain food products is that, just like the tobacco companies in the early seventies, they are fully aware these products are not going to help people lose weight and get healthy. Not only is it not going to help them, but nine times out of ten it will exacerbate the problem – gits!

ENRICHED

Then you have the 'enriched with vitamins and minerals', the 'added calcium' and the 'fortified with...' labels. Once again you can't just add processed, totally de-natured vitamins and calcium and expect them to make a drug food good – because they just won't. The biggest beef I have with them is that they imply they are doing you a favour by adding these things and enriching your food. Don't forget the only reason why it was poor to begin with was because of them and the only thing they are enriching is their bank accounts.

It seems strange to me that it is perfectly legal to buy 'organic', 'GM free', 'no artificial colour', 'fat-free' white refined pasta. This all combines to give the very false impression that you are buying a health food. But who cares if it's organic, GM free or has no artificial colourings? IT'S STILL A WHITE REFINED DRUG-LIKE FOOD and as such is so far from a health food that it's a joke. Can you imagine if the tobacco companies started to sell organically-grown, GM-free, no artificial colouring, vitamin-enriched, all-natural, fat-free, low-calorie, light, added calcium and fortified with vitamin C cigarettes? Would it make any difference? No, because they would still contain nicotine, which is the drug that compels people to have more and more, and keeps them enslaved. And exactly the same principle applies to drug-like foods. The white refined sugars and carbs are like the nicotine of the food world.

The only way to free yourself from the food trap is first to understand the nature of what we are dealing with, then to use the mental tools which will enable you to actually quit the rubbish, change brands, eat plenty of food and get mentally and physically juiced. Please remember you do not yet have the mental juice or tools that will guarantee your freedom for life – we are in fact still on the first stage of understanding the trap. I will show you how to *think* (the mental juice) very soon, but it really would be meaningless to do it now without a *full* understanding of the food trap and how they will do anything, from creating 'bells' and false advertising to blatantly putting misleading words and statements on their products.

And please bear in mind they don't just do this with food either. A major part of the 'food' industry's revenue comes not from what people eat, but from what they drink. And they use all the same false advertising, misleading labels, and *physical* drug-like substances to keep you hooked. So let us raise our glasses to an anything but…

20

Liquid Asset

Water, water everywhere and not a drop to drink

I think that anyone who is reading this book is already aware that our bodies need water and plenty of it. The planet is, after all, made up of over 70 per cent of the stuff and so too are our bodies. All foods which were clearly meant for human consumption also contain at least 70 per cent water. Even a banana, which you would imagine contains very little, is over 80 per cent water. There is not one single fruit or veg meant for us that contains less than 80 per cent water – a bit of a clue methinks. The water that fruit provides can be described as a true 'liquid asset', as it has the added advantage of having bundles of live nutrients flowing through it. These replenish your body's bank accounts, making it feel light and flowing with energy, and much less susceptible to disease.

However, the majority of liquid going down most people's gullets is a far cry from an asset – certainly not the high-caffeine coffee and tea we seem to 'need' several times daily or the caffeine- and sugar-laced 'soft' drinks that are earning billions for the food industry, yet in turn helping to put our magnificent industry (the body) into liquidation. And once again the only reason why people continue to drink these fat-producing, calcium-robbing, insulin-pumping 'soft' drinks, even when they know they're bad for them, is the usual cocktail of brain-washing advertisements and addictive ingredients.

The advertising for what I describe as drug drinks is even bigger than that for drug foods. They are, of course, bound to make more money out of drug drinks as they not only create withdrawal symptoms and low blood sugar to keep you hooked, but they are also designed to *cause* dehydration. And as they don't fill the stomach, there is no cut-off point. Which all means it's very easy for them to convince us that it is, once again, our genuine choice to drink these substances. But if you feel dehydrated you don't have a choice, you must drink. These drinks, like alcohol, are cleverly designed to cause the dehydration you believe you are getting rid of with the drug drink. At the same time, if you are in a constant state of withdrawal (from caffeine for example) or your sugar levels are beginning to crash because of your white sugar addiction, then you are certainly going to feel a sense of satisfaction and pleasure – first from the liquid, then from the partial ending of the caffeine withdrawal and finally, from bringing your sugar levels back up. The combination of all of this gives the very strong feeling of pleasure. But again, as with any drug, the pleasure is simply the ending of an aggravation, mental and physical, which has been caused by the drug itself. In this case you have three aggravations in one, all seemingly being satisfied with an instant fix of the drug drink. So the relief the body feels will be quite immense, which gives you an instant feeling of pleasure, an instant rush that makes you believe you are choosing to drink this muck. But I cannot repeat this point enough, it's not a *genuine* pleasure, it is a false one and is the equivalent of carrying around a heavy boulder just to get the pleasure of putting it down every now and then! In such circumstances you would feel better, but why pick it up in the first place?

The problem is that you have been carrying around the boulder for so long you can't even feel it any more. You now believe this is a normal way to feel, you think it's just life and the usual stresses and strains that are dragging you down – not the boulder. And because nearly everyone you meet feels the same, you believe it must be normal. But it's not normal – you are waking up with a drug food and drug drink hangover every single day. How do you instantly solve this problem? An instant drug food and drug drink lift. These foods and drinks *appear* to be your best friends: life's knocking you down, but at least you can always rely on your coffee and muffins (or whatever) to help pick you up. But the more you try and lift yourself up with these types of drinks or foods the hangover will *always* get just that little bit worse. When it does you either have to use willpower, discipline or control not to increase your intake, or give in to it and increase the dose. But you are still using the very things that are causing you to feel like crap on a consistent basis. This is why people have such difficulty changing their eating and drinking habits – they feel as though they're losing a friend and hence experience a sense of loss. That sense of loss is often just too much to bear and results in a feeling of emptiness. What do most people turn to when they feel empty and alone? A friend. If you believe that these drug foods and drinks are your friends and will actually *solve* the way you are feeling you will 'give in' and the whole cycle starts again. That is why people struggle when they try to quit certain drug foods or drug drinks. It's not the withdrawal from the drug that is the problem, but the belief that you get something from them. We need to first remove the belief, then get rid of the drug-like foods and drinks.

The mini hangovers caused by drug drinks are, as previously mentioned, seemingly solved by the instant physical reaction you feel when having a drug drink fix. This alone can easily delude you into a set of false beliefs which keep you hooked. However, on top of this you once again have the massive amount of advertising that seems to reinforce the false impression of the thirst-quenching, energy-boosting and, of course, pleasure-giving qualities of these drinks.

The two major players in the drug drink war are Pepsi and Coke and these two have been battling for years to get the biggest market share. Ad after ad, one product placement after another, they will do anything and say anything to get you to switch to their brand of drug drink. The main market share is once again children; 1 in 8 of whom are now consuming **22 cans of cola each week – yes 22 cans**! As a nation we get through 8–10,000 million litres of 'soft' drinks every year, and that number is constantly on the increase. But I wonder how much Coke, Pepsi or any other 'soft' drink they would sell if by law they had to tell the truth and do some 'truthful' advertising?

'Buy Coke. It contains 6–7 teaspoons of white refined sugar – almost guaranteed to hook ya. And in case it doesn't, we've added highly addictive caffeine with the sole purpose of making it habit-forming – just to make sure we've got ya as a sucker, I mean customer, for life. And let's not forget the phosphoric acid – something so toxic and dangerous that if you put enamel into it, it would dissolve it. If that's not enough, we've made sure that the acid effect on your body will rob calcium from your bones and teeth, while the sugar will cause tons of the fat-producing hormone insulin to be secreted – which is guaranteed to overwork your pancreas. Plus the added white refined sugar will coat your teeth like nothing else and the beautiful tasty phosphoric acid will help to dissolve them. So please, as our slogan has read for years...

HAVE A COKE AND A SMILE

If you are still able to that is. I want to make it clear here I am not simply talking about Coke, I am talking about virtually *all* 'soft' drinks. If Coke had no competition they wouldn't even need to advertise. A few fixes of the drug drink and you're hooked; you would buy it anyway. The only reason why they all advertise drug drinks over and over again is because they *all* contain the same addictive and health-destroying shit, but if they can convince you their brand is 'cooler' or tastier you will switch – and that's all they want.

All of these drug drinks either contain loads of caffeine, massive quantities of white trashy sugar or a combination of the two. These substances are the nicotine of the drug drink world. That's without mentioning the acids, colourings, flavourings and so on which each can is also loaded with.

As I've said, it's not just Coke and Pepsi that are playing the keep 'em hooked game, they're all at it. From Dr Pepper trying to convince us all he is 'so misunderstood', being slapped on the head or 'Tangoed', Lilt with its totally tropical taste, to the Sprite boys trying to tell us that they have no intention of selling glamour with their drink – it's all about 'obeying your thirst'. The last one has more than a touch of irony as the white refined sugar and some of the other rubbish you find swimming about in it causes a degree of dehydration. Then there's

Lucozade which, when I was growing up, was marketed for sick people. If anyone was ill the first thing you bought them was a big bottle of Lucozade. Wow what a 'bell' – they managed to convince an entire population that if you were ill it would be of benefit to drink some Lucozade. Their slogan even seemed to back-up what they were saying and in turn our beliefs about it: 'Lucozade aids recovery'. Some doctors were even recommending this stuff to their already sick patients. This stuff contains white refined sugar, flavourings, colourings and preservatives – oh, and 5 per cent fruit juice.

Some manufacturers have launched a new breed of 'stimulating', 'vitalizing', 'boosting', 'energy-giving' drinks which I consider is just the latest way to market liquid drugs to a new generation. These drinks actually claim to 'increase physical endurance', 'improve and increase concentration and reaction speed', 'lift you' and 'give you an energy rush'. There is only one thing I have to say about them –

Total bull (usually of the red kind)

Yes indeed, Red Bull, or rather Red 'total' Bull as I call it. 'It gives you wings don't ya know' – their words not mine. What the hell are they banging on about – it gives you wings. What does? And it's not only Red Bull, there are plenty of companies that have joined the 'boost' drink bandwagon. You have 'Power Horse' (wow what a name), 'Dynamite' and a few others like them claiming similar nonsense. They were always onto a sure bet too with these kinds of drinks as most of their customers are waking up every day with a degree of drug food or drug drink hangover (or a combination of the two). The more wiped out people feel, the more 'energy boosting' drinks they sell: their need for 'wings', a lift in other words, becomes greater by the day. Red Bull and the like contain a lot, and I mean a lot, of caffeine – more than Coke that's for sure and enough to make the French ban the drink altogether in early 2004. One small can of Solstis contains the same amount as one cup of coffee. They also contain loads of white refined sugar or 'glucose syrup' as they put it.

So what's going to happen again? Withdrawal and low blood sugar – the body has an abnormal boost and in no time hits a low. The more lows felt the greater the need for the boost. The more you boost the lower you get, the lower you get the more you need the boost. You end up playing catch up – simply trying to get to where you were before you started having them. This is exactly how all drugs work.

IT'S ISOTONIC

Another energy drink, Lucozade Sport, claims: 'In tests against water, athletes using Lucozade Sport drinks are proven to improve their sporting performance by 33 per cent. Why? Sport scientists have proved that depletion of carbohydrate energy stores and fluid impair performance. Lucozade Sport is *isotonic* – it's specially formulated to be in balance with your body's own fluid. It quickly delivers a boost of carbohydrate energy to the working muscles and supplies fluid fast, which together help to maximize performance and endurance.'

Here's the thing – SO DOES FRUIT. I could make exactly the same claim about fruit, as it would enable you to go on longer than water alone – but then you don't need to be Inspector Morse to work that one out do you? Look at what they actually say, 'Sports scientists have proved that depletion of carbohydrate energy stores and fluid impair performance'. Do you think they worked that one out by themselves? OF COURSE IT WOULD, as we'd then lack two of our basic requirements – water and carbs (fuel). If you replace them you will of course improve performance and endurance. If you are an athlete be assured there's simply no better form of carb energy than humble fruit – just ask Tim Henman. Like drug foods, drug drinks sometimes do the complete opposite to what we are led to believe they will.

Red Bull and isotonic sports drinks are not the only new players in the drug drink game, and they are far from being the only ones to promote their product as in some way good for you. There is, however, one drug drink which is, in my opinion, the most sinister of the entire lot. I am talking here about a drink that just seemed to spring out of nowhere. One day the supermarket fridges were full of 'freshly squeezed' orange juice and the next they were full of Sunny Delight – it was everywhere. I thought it was unusual to have such a heavy push for fresh orange juice – until I read the label!

SUNNY DE-FRIGHT

The front of the label shows a big bright sun and of course the words
Sunny Delight. In the corner it reads: 'The great taste of 4 fruits with
5 vitamins. Vitamins A-B (1&6) C-E enriched beverage.' Given this
wording, and the fact the stuff is displayed in the 'fruit juice' fridges, I
strongly suspect people are convinced that what they're buying is a
healthy, vitamin-packed fruit juice – WRONG. You are in fact buying a
bottle of highly-sugared, chemical-laced liquid which contains just 5
per cent fruit juice. Let me say that again – *5 per cent fruit juice.*
The thing which really angers me about this particular product is that
the advertising is not only aimed at children (as is the case for many
drug drinks) but the marketers deliberately set out to convince
parents that they were buying a 'healthy' juice drink for their kids.
Parents who tell their kids that Coke and Pepsi are a 'no-no' are letting
them have Sunny Delight with impunity. The number of people I see in
my seminars who think Sunny Delight is just a fruit juice is scary. The
fact is that it contains so much sugar that it doesn't even need to be
kept in the fridge and the sell by date is always months down the line.
Parents are not stupid for thinking Sunny Delight is good for their
kids – they are made to believe it. The makers will, of course, argue
that they do tell us on the label, but the true info is in small print on
the back. These people are peddling drug drinks on children and
bloody shame on them – how they sleep at night I just don't know.
The money comforts them, I guess. So successful was their £9m
advertising campaign for this liquid frightener that sales topped
£150m a year.

If you think my views about certain members of the drug drink
industry are somewhat over-the-top, please remember that I deal with
the long-term effects of this kind of manipulation every day from
people who are often very desperate to kick their sugar addiction.
People whose excess weight is affecting every single area of their
lives; people whose organs are packing up; people who are having to
inject themselves with insulin every single day because their bank
account has run out; and people who live with – and often don't know
what to with – their hyperactive children. This is why I name the stuff

Sunny De*fright*, because the short- and long-term effects of sugar addiction can be very frightening indeed.

The drug drink industry will literally stop at nothing to get your money and keep you as a customer for life – regardless of the cost to your body or sanity. Their problem is that the stuff they are pushing rots teeth, helps to weaken bones and – more importantly for most people – makes them fat. And customers were beginning to recognize this. So what did companies like Coke and Pepsi do? They brought out diet versions of their highly toxic drug drinks in an attempt to make people believe that if they switch to the diet brands it would help them lose weight. It worked, millions believed it – I was one of them.

These diet drinks are deliberately marketed to give you the impression they are in some way healthy and, of course, their main aim is to make you believe they will help you to lose weight. The truth is you have about as much chance of getting healthy and losing weight with the help of these products as getting run over by a number 12 bus going up the side of Ben Nevis with Ronald Reagan at the wheel!

The sad fact is they conditioned and hooked us so much on 'normal' Coke and Pepsi that we thought it was good when they came out with a non-fattening alternative. However, the nightmare substances to be found in the diet versions, combined with the fact we believe them to be non-fattening, means we end up drinking more of them than the 'real' stuff anyway. Of all the substances I talk about, one of the very worst is to be found in virtually *all* diet drinks. It's one which I believe is reason enough to give yourself a true…

21

Diet Coke Break

Ah yes, Diet Coke, the drink which – and please listen carefully – 'Can help you lose weight as part of a calorie controlled diet'. Guess what, reading a newspaper can also help you lose weight – *as part of a calorie controlled diet*! I want to make it clear – anything that is toxic to the body is not going to make it healthy nor is it going to help it to lose weight healthily. How they get away with this type of claptrap is a complete mystery. It becomes even more of a mystery when you hear of the many problems which have been linked to diet drinks and foods.

There is only one reason why people drink diet drinks – they are 'sugar free' and as such the hope is it will stop them getting fat. But there is now strong evidence to suggest these diet drinks and foods actually contribute to weight *gain*. Let me say that again –

There is strong evidence to suggest that diet foods and drinks can actually make you fat

The one ingredient common to all these 'sugar-free' drinks and foods is the chemical aspartame, also known as E951 and better known under the brand names of Nutrasweet and Canderel. Aspartame was discovered accidentally by the chemist James Schlatter back in 1969.

He was testing a new chemical as a possible anti-ulcer drug when some of the liquid went on his hand. When he licked it he discovered a gold mine – it tasted incredibly sweet. In fact aspartame is over 200 times sweeter than sugar yet contains virtually no calories – bingo! He just knew he was onto a massive financial winner.

However, it took 16 years for US drug giant Searle (his company) to win FDA approval for the sweetener. In 1981 an internal memo from three FDA scientists advised *against* the approval of aspartame. Yet in exactly the same year Ronald Reagan, then president, fired the FDA commissioner and a Dr Arthur Hull Hayes inherited the job. Just three months later aspartame was passed for *limited* use and within two years was allowed in drinks. The floodgates were open and many countries followed suit. These days aspartame is found in just about every 'sugar free' food and drink you can think of. It's even found its way into sugar free gum, baby foods and chewable vitamin tablets.

So why was the FDA so against it for so long? Because aspartame has been linked to 92 different symptoms including headaches, skin problems, poor vision, depression, carbohydrate cravings, panic attacks, irregular heart rhythms, behavioural problems, seizures and most worrying of all – brain tumours. One senior FDA toxicologist said,

'At least one test has established beyond any reasonable doubt that aspartame is capable of producing brain tumours in animals'

Your brain is normally protected by something called the blood-brain barrier; a safety net that usually prevents harmful substances passing from the blood to the brain. The problem is that aspartame is believed by many to damage the hypothalamus – the area of the brain responsible for regulating the emotional control system, the hormonal and reproductive systems, appetite, immunity and memory. It is worth noting that this area of the brain is not protected by the blood-brain barrier – hence the possible link to brain tumours. This could also be why headaches are a very common symptom for many aspartame users. The surgeon general, head of the public health service in the US, said they believe aspartame usage to be a *major contributing factor* to the 22 million Americans who suffer from mental disorders.

Dr Hyman Roberts for the Palm Beach Institute for Medical Research in Florida, initially welcomed aspartame: 'When it was introduced, I recommended it to diabetic patients because it contained no sugar, calories, cholesterol or sodium. I thought it was a godsend.' But he had second thoughts after more and more patients developed problems such as chronic headaches, impaired vision and panic attacks. He soon narrowed down the culprit to aspartame. Around 1200 patients reported an adverse reaction to this nightmare substance, the most common being headaches. Dr Roberts added, 'I have also had numerous diabetic patients whose condition has been exacerbated by aspartame, including eye and nerve problems. However, when they were taken off aspartame they improved dramatically'. His findings are supported by those of Dr Russell Blaylock, a Missouri neurosurgeon who has what he sees as conclusive proof that aspartame causes terrible changes in behaviour. He says, 'My advice is if you are consuming products containing aspartame, stop using them for three weeks and see for yourself the dramatic difference in the way you feel'.

I believe the main problem is that far from solving weight problems – which it kind of claims to do and is the only reason people buy the stuff – it is suggested by many that it actually causes overeating. Here's why. Aspartame seems to impede the production of the chemical serotonin and a lack of serotonin is not only widely believed to cause depression and mood disorders, but is also linked to such eating disorders as binge eating. This kind of defeats the whole object of diet drinks somewhat don't you think? Dr Ralph Walton, professor at the department of psychiatry at Northeast Ohio University's College of Medicine, believes the calorie-saving advantage of aspartame is totally thwarted because it makes people prone to binge eating. He even says, 'If you feed a laboratory animal aspartame, you wind up with an obese animal'. His advice to those trying to slim is pretty clear:

'...if you are trying to lose weight, you should stay away from aspartame'.

He is not alone either. Betty Martini, a leading US food safety campaigner, is equally scathing. 'We see literally thousands of cases of people who have been taking aspartame for a long time, and they are *always* overweight. Aspartame actually makes you crave carbohydrates so that you *gain* weight'.

Aspartame also dehydrates the body, creating a greater need for fluid. You can physically only drink a certain amount of water before the body tells you it's had enough, but with diet drinks you can consume one after another and still feel thirsty.

As you can see there are plenty of reasons to avoid this stuff. But, as always, be your own scientist. If you have drunk diet drinks for years and are still fat what more proof do you need? Diet drinks are equally as bad as the original version, if not worse, so once again the manufacturers are having a laugh at our expense. They get us fat with the original versions, by making them addictive and bombarding us with misleading advertising, and then sell us over 5 billion cans of the diet versions a year, which can make us binge eat, crave carbs, dehydrate our bodies and still keep us fat! Diet Tango's slogan is 'you need it cos you're weak' – how's that for saying up yours? That's like a cigarette company saying you need cigarettes because you're weak, but you become weak *because* of cigarettes and you need them because you're hooked. And the same goes for sugar, caffeine and aspartame.

If nothing else, even if you don't make any other change, do yourself and your kids a huge favour by breaking free from aspartame or any other 'sweetener'. These drinks don't help you to get slim, they don't genuinely quench your thirst, they don't help to reduce your intake of the wrong kinds of food – if anything they do the complete opposite. Once you have some juice power pumping through your veins you just won't feel the need to constantly drink something as the juice will *genuinely* quench your thirst and furnish your body with the fluid it thrives on.

DRUNK BLIND

Most people are drinking these drug-like chemical concoctions blindly: blinded by what I believe to be misleading advertising, misleading packaging and the false sense of pleasure received by the partial ending of the very mental and physical aggravations *they* cause. I call it the 'drunk blind' syndrome – when you are drinking something blindly, not able to see the truth. Once you can see clearly what's going on you become free *not* to drink them; until then you remain hooked.

All of the drug foods and drug drinks mentioned thus far play their part in knocking you down. The further down you go, the more you want a quick 'pick me up'. The irony is when you get rid of these nightmare foods and drinks from your life you won't need a 'pick-me-up' because you will already be up. The only reason why people continue with the loop is to try and get to the position they could be in if only they didn't eat or drink them.

The most common and most widely used 'pick-me-ups' of them all – and ones which are so ingrained into our culture that 98 per cent of people in the UK drink them several times daily – are our old friends coffee and tea. Now, as everyone knows, you don't have to give these up in order to get slim BUT if you want to *calm* your nervous system, *calm* your mind, keep your looks and tap into a level of physical and mental vibrancy you never thought possible it's time for your…

22

Coffee Wake up Call

Yep, it's time to wake up and smell the coffee – whilst you think twice about actually drinking the stuff. This is one addiction people strongly believe is difficult to break, but the reality is that it's actually easy. If you don't think you need a break from coffee or tea, I can assure you your body is screaming for one. In fact it's worth pointing out that if the amount of caffeine found in just a single cup of coffee were injected directly into your bloodstream it would kill you. The good news, however, is that caffeine only takes a maximum of 48 hours to leave your body completely and the physical pain you have to suffer because of this is in reality nil – especially when you have plenty of Juice Master juice replacing lost fluid.

The struggle people have when trying to 'give up' coffee and tea is not a physical one – just like all drug foods and drinks, the struggle is mental. The UK is the only place on earth where if a war breaks out people say, 'I'll put the kettle on'. These drug drinks are used as emotional crutches. This is why many people will stop putting sugar in their coffee or tea, or maybe cut down slightly on them, but get rid of them completely – not on your Nelly!

Most people assume they will still get slim as long as they cut out the sugar. However, I strongly suggest a total tea and coffee break for the following reasons. You may not gain weight directly because of tea or coffee, but both shatter the central nervous system, cause with-drawal lows and, in the long run, make you even more tired. This has a knock-on effect, causing lethargy in the mind, a restlessness in the body and ultimately more 'Oh sod it' moods in your day. These 'sod it' moods cause you to overeat drug and junk foods. So although they don't directly cause weight problems, they indirectly play their part in keeping you well below your natural, vibrant best. Having said that, caffeine does cause the stomach to produce gastric acid, which stimulates your appetite.

There is also simply no other liquid drug drink which speeds up the ageing process quicker than caffeine, and most people get their daily dose through coffee, tea and Coke (or more recently Red Bull). People are spending billions on external creams and lotions to 'fight the ageing process', 'to slow down the signs of ageing'. But why waste your money; you can't *slow down* the ageing process. You can, however, do a million different things to speed it up – and drinking caffeine on a regular basis is one of the best ways to do just that. Many people don't realize this because compared to most people they look okay and are ageing no faster than the majority of people around them. But the majority of people around them are eating drug foods and drinking drug drinks the same as them, all of which speed up the ageing of every single organ in the body.

YOU'RE GETTING ON MY NERVES

People often say, 'I feel like I'm living on my nerves' and the sad reality is they very often are. Every time you drink a cup of coffee or tea (or a Coke or Red Bull), you jolt your nervous system and dehydrate your body. It's like being in a constant state of stress – your kidneys and liver take a battering, you overwork your adrenal glands and you rob your body and brain of water. Caffeine is a strong diuretic – meaning it makes you pee. This all helps to *speed up* the ageing process and literally makes your nerves stand on end. Not only that but if you keep dehydrating your body the kidneys will conserve water by making less urine. As a result of this the urine becomes highly concentrated which leads to crystals separating out. These crystals can eventually build up and produce KIDNEY STONES. I think I'll pass on that thank you.

The dehydration also affects the brain. Your brain is made up of mainly water and when you are in a state of caffeine withdrawal you lose some of it. Now your brain is smaller than it was – which I guess shatters the notion that coffee helps you to concentrate. (But then I couldn't concentrate properly if I was withdrawing from a drug either.) Blood still has to pump through your brain in order to keep you alive. And when blood is pumping through a dehydrated brain you feel it pounding inside your skull – commonly known as a headache. On top of this you also have caffeine withdrawal which makes your nervous system feel insecure – in turn making you feel jittery. So with your head pounding, your mouth as dry as the Sahara desert and your nerves in tatters what do you reach for? A nice cup of coffee.

The problem is when you drink it what happens? YOU DO FEEL BETTER, that's why you reached for it. If you didn't there would be no hook. I cannot repeat enough that what hooks people on these drug foods and drinks is not so much the substance itself, but what you *think* the substance is doing for you. The drug-like foods and drinks are ultimately to blame because they have managed to delude us into believing we get some sort of genuine pleasure and relief from them. Once you have more coffee you have put more fluid into the body which helps with the pounding head and dehydration, you partially end your withdrawal from the drug itself and your nervous system actually feels calmer than it did. This all combines to make us think the opposite to what is actually happening – we are deluded into believing that the coffee helped, as opposed to *caused*, the situation. Unless you know that it was the caffeine which helped to cause these problems you will play catch-up all your life and *never* get there. It is the delusion which hooks us.

'BUT IT'S NICE TO HAVE A COFFEE BREAK'

Yes and smokers think it's nice to have a cigarette break and crack-heads think it's nice to have a crack break. The point is it's just nice to have a break – period. You don't need to shove something down your throat at the same time to enjoy a break. When a smoker is having a 'break', they will stand outside on a fire escape in the middle of a hurricane. Do they do this for fun? To be sociable? No, they do it because they are drug addicts. Exactly the same principle applies to coffee – the only difference is that it is not considered unsociable and you don't have to stand outside in a hurricane to have your fix.

These drink drugs knock the nervous system so much that the person drinking them is made to believe that they won't be able to cope properly with life or even wake up without the stuff. Tea and coffee have such a mental link because they tend to be drunk at nice *times*, such as when people come round, breaks from work, getting in after a hard day etc. I like coming home after a hard day too, but the difference is that I don't need drug foods or drinks to help me relax any more for one reason – my nervous system is now *already* relaxed. People are trying to relax themselves or 'lift' themselves with the very substances that are causing their nervous system to feel jittery and their bodies tired.

Dr David Kerr of the Royal Bournemouth Hospital summed it up when he said, 'Within half an hour of drinking one or two cups, the flow of blood to the brain is reduced by 10–20 per cent. Combine that with low blood sugar and you can soon start to have palpitations, feelings of anxiety or blurred vision'. And that's just one or two cups. The average is over six, which is a nightmare for your nervous system. Please also bear in mind that when caffeine hits the central nervous system it *lowers* blood sugar, which *increases* the brain's demand for more sugar. Let me repeat that in case you skimmed by it –

When caffeine hits the central nervous system it lowers blood sugar and increases the brain's demand for sugar

This, in turn, helps to keep people rooted in the food trap. It is also worth noting that every time you drink tea and coffee our old friend insulin is released, once again helping to batter the pancreas.

So am I saying you can never have a cup of tea or coffee again? No, you can do as you please. I'm just pointing out that they don't do what you think and the pleasure you get is just the relief from withdrawal. In other words you get nothing from them apart from mental and physical abuse. And if you think you only drink coffee for the taste of it, then why is the thought of getting rid of it so scary? You wouldn't feel the same if you were told you had to give up a particularly delicious fruit you love. So why do people panic when they think about getting rid of drug foods and drug drinks like coffee? Because they all undermine the central nervous system and batter your confidence to the point where they make you believe your life wouldn't be the same without them. And coffee and tea are two of the most widely used drug drinks which seem to have everyone fooled. Places like Starbucks are no doubt well aware of the mental addiction people have for coffee. The more it knocks them down the more they seemingly need to restore them to any shred of normality. This is why, in the US in particular, you see queues of caffeine junkies waiting in the cold for their first fix of the day. This is not choice – it's slavery to a drink drug. This is borne out by the fact that coffee is now the second most legally traded commodity in the world – the first is oil. The stats on this stuff are quite staggering: 60 per cent of Britons are said to visit the new 'hip' generation of coffee shops once or twice a day – that adds up to a hell of a lot of revenue, as you will discover later.

CUP OF FORMALDEHYDE ANYONE?

Now I'm not saying that everyone who goes and grabs a Starbucks is hooked on the stuff and I'm not saying that you cannot have the odd cup of tea or coffee and still be slim and healthy, because clearly you can. But if you *are* hooked (and you'll know who you are) then it's worth knowing that there are plenty of non-addictive alternatives to tea and coffee, which, once you've adjusted, are actually nicer and more satisfying. I now drink all kinds of teas, from peppermint to camomile, but my fave is simply some hot water with a slice of lemon or lime in it (don't knock it 'till you've tried it!). One thing I'm certainly not recommending as an alternative though is decaf tea or coffee. Once again, the product which they market as a 'healthy' alternative is anything but. First of all, decaffeinated coffee still has some caffeine in it (how they get away with that is again a mystery). Secondly, two of the chemicals used to decaffeinate coffee are turpentine and formaldehyde. Formaldehyde is used as an embalming fluid – lovely!

But remember all drug drinks and drug-like foods have no other hold over you than what you *believe* you get from them – once you see the truth, the belief is changed and freedom is yours for the taking. It really can be that simple. And when you do free yourself of these substances you won't believe how much calmer and more relaxed you become.

Unfortunately the truth is not always easy to see. The clever advertising, the product placements, the misinformation we have had from the experts since birth and, of course, the constant *illusory* 'boosts' caused by the drug-like substances all combine to keep us from seeing the truth that will set us free. And because these substances shatter and jolt the nervous system – making our lives *appear* a lot more stressful than they really are – this can have the knock-on effect of making us turn to yet another drug drink. The one I am talking about here makes it very difficult to see the truth. In fact it makes it very difficult to see – full stop. It is so ingrained in our society that if you don't *drink* it, you are questioned as to why and viewed as having a problem with it. Yet it's a drug drink which is responsible for more deaths, more violence, more suicides, more break-ups, more domestic violence, more child abuse and more heartache than crack, cocaine, LSD, ecstasy and heroin combined. It is a substance which is just as toxic as heroin, yet parents seem quite happy to give this substance to their children – often before they've reached double figures. This drug drink not only piles on the pounds, due to its toxicity, but also messes with your mind and creates overwhelming cravings for carbohydrates and sugars. It not only causes you to overeat at times but has also been known to distort the mind so much that people have been known to eat things they would never normally touch whilst under its influence. That was perhaps the biggest clue because, let's face facts, when it comes to food, anything looks good when you are literally...

23

Blind Drunk

Time please ladies and gentlemen – for an eye opener

'Okay Jason I was with you right up until now. Getting shot of Coke, tea and cheese is one thing, but if you think I am quitting my glass of wine with dinner or the odd beer when I'm out with the lads or lasses – forget it pal. This is meant to be a lifestyle and not a diet and I have no intention of going without alcohol for the rest of my life. I am not an alcoholic, I do not have a drink problem, so why should I?'

Well if that's how you are thinking you'll be relieved to hear that you do not have to quit alcohol altogether in order to have a slim, energy-driven body. But it certainly is worth looking at this highly toxic, fat-producing substance with our eyes very much wide open. This can only happen when we are sober for when we are drunk, we really do become totally blind. Blind to our feelings, blind to our emotions, blind to our behaviour, blind to what's going on around us and totally blind to what we are actually putting into our body – and I don't simply mean the insulin-robbing, fat-producing alcohol. We need to open our eyes and realize it's not just the alcohol that piles on the pounds, batters our organs, acts as a depressant, causes lethargy, keeps us a slave and helps to once again speed up the ageing process; it's also the crap we eat because of it.

I believe alcohol came first, kebabs second. Kebabs really do fit into the 'mystery food' category: big chunks of 'whatever-the-hell-it-is' meat, stuffed into a white refined pitta, the token salad (if you can ever describe it as such), topped off with blow-your-head-off chilli sauce (why is it called chilli?). You see this big mound of flesh hanging up in a warm shop window for what seems like months. As you walk past during the day, neither hell nor high water could get you put that putrefying lump of dead flesh into your mouth. Just the thought of the flies laying their eggs and defecating on it (as they do when they land on food) is normally enough to keep any rational, thinking person well away. But I did say rationally-thinking person and any kind of reason or thinking goes completely out of the window when you're a couple of jars short of a coma. In fact, when you come piling out of your local pub or nightclub this lump of fly-poo-infested mystery food magically turns into the finest gourmet cuisine. And it's not only kebabs. These are also the times when the 'hot mystery food' van – which on the way into the nightclub was just a rotting old dirty van with a big fat scruffy dribbley man attempting to serve you rubbish – all of a sudden becomes heaven on wheels.

The alcohol is devastating enough for your bloodstream – the last thing it needs is a load of blood-clogging, fat-laden, sugar-infested 'food' seeping through it at the same time. But what choice do you have when you're drunk? You've lost your normal control, your sugar levels are out of sync, and your body has been stripped of essential fats, vitamins and minerals – which all add up to an unbelievable craving for something stodgy to try and satisfy the empty feeling.

The body now has so much poison going into it that it needs to shut down in order to keep you alive. Once again it calls on eyesight, hearing and whatever consciousness is left to help it out with this red alert situation. The problem is so bad that the body just doesn't have the energy to keep you alive and awake at the same time – so it shuts down. You are now in a comatose state that even beats the Christmas dinner one. The body has such a need to repair itself that even if someone was to pick you up by the feet, swing you around the room and through the window – you still wouldn't wake up. No, the only thing governing whether you are allowed any form of consciousness is your body, and quite frankly it just has too much work to do and needs all the energy it can muster.

There is, however, one point at which the body will allow you to get up and move – when it either needs to release fluid or when it calls for fluid. If the situation is particularly bad the body may not even wake you up to release fluid – it will just do it. Sometimes, of course, it may compromise with you by allowing you to get up and move but not giving you any sense of direction – this is when you end up releasing bodily fluid either in the wrong room or in the cupboard! However, when the body wants fluid it will certainly wake you up and make you move as fast as you can to replenish lost fluid. Ah yes, the 'Sahara Desert Syndrome' as I call it. This is where you wake up in the middle of the night with what can only be described as the mother of all thirsts. The body is so dehydrated that unless it gets some water – soon – you are in a serious danger of either dying or at least causing some kind of brain damage. So the body calls to the brain 'WAKE UP AND GIVE ME SOME WATER NOW'. This is the point where we sit bolt upright in bed (if we ever made it there), trying to catch our breath through an extremely dry throat. Now it's sod the 'I only drink mineral water' nonsense – where's the nearest tap? Once the body can't hold any more water without bursting, it orders you back to sleep – not rest, sleep. After all, your body is hardly resting is it? So back in a coma we go. We eventually wake up to find that the Royal Philharmonic Orchestra has set up temporary residence inside our skull and our body feels like it's been run over by a truck.

So what's really going on here? Well your brain is now smaller than it was the night before – it has literally shrunk. I just want to say that again –

Your brain is smaller than it was the night before

The water you lose because of the massive dehydrating effect of alcohol causes this. Have you ever noticed that for every beer you drink you tend to pee out three? Water is the next thing the body needs after oxygen to function efficiently. Without it you will wither and die. Every single cell and organ relies on it, including the all important head office – your brain. That little bit of water you had during the night helped a bit, but your brain (which is mainly water) is still very dehydrated – this makes it shrink in size. Every time you have a skinful it's like going into the ring with Mike Tyson. Alcohol destroys brain cells, did you know that? If the brain is constantly (like a few times a week for example) deprived of water to this extent and is at the same time beaten up by the highly toxic alcohol – it can easily cause *permanent* shrinkage and damage to the brain. When you wake up with your brain shrunk on say a Sunday morning (the most common time) blood still has to pump through it in order to keep you alive. The pounding feeling in your head is no less than blood trying to pump through a dehydrated brain. Your head hurts like hell, your body feels weak and one more thing, your blood sugar levels – which govern hunger – are very, very low. This causes a massive empty feeling and a mother of a hunger. You see it's not just the alcohol that's the problem, or even the crap mystery food we eat when we are drunk, but also the rubbish we crave when we wake up with a stonker of a hangover.

First up, it's the painkillers. Excellent – this is about the last thing your body needs. These tablets don't get rid of a headache; they just move the ache or cover it up. What do I mean? When you put a painkiller into your system it simply shuts off nerve endings to your brain. So you still have blood trying to pump through a dehydrated brain, only now you've taken a painkiller you can't feel it any more. But just because you can't feel it doesn't mean it's not happening. And because you have now buggered up your body's *natural* action signals, you will ignore your body's calls for what it really needs – rest, nutrients and FLUID.

So with the headache apparently sorted, what's next? Ah yes, the blood sugar levels which have crashed to an all-week low. When your sugar levels crash to that extent you crave an instant fix – and broccoli just ain't going to do it. You need something that's going to raise your sugar levels *quickly*. You have such an empty feeling that you feel the need to load your bloodstream with sugar and fats – ASAP. So you crave fry-ups, white refined bread, croissants, jam, salt etc. All this drug-like food comes flooding into an already battered and very tired body. It's difficult enough for the body to try and process rubbish food like this normally, but with alcohol in the system – fat chance, literally. Alcohol is so toxic to the body that it cannot be stored anywhere; the body must get rid of it as soon as it can or it will die. This means that while the body is dealing with the alcohol it leaves anything you've eaten the night before or that morning untouched. This all adds up to the type of 'hang over' which can be with you for a long time – yes the very uncomfortable 'flesh hang over' commonly known as fat.

And we try to counteract this type of hangover by mixing some *Diet Coke* with the fat-producing alcohol – as if adding Diet Coke to our 10 vodkas is really going to make any difference to our weight or energy levels. We not only mix aspartame with alcohol, but we also mix the new 'energy' drinks with them too – probably to try and counter the effect of the alcohol. A hip drink at the moment is vodka mixed with our old friend Red Bull. So here we have a depressant (alcohol) and a stimulant (Red Bull) in the same glass – no wonder we don't know if we're coming or going. Now if we go by one of the many myths about alcohol, you shouldn't ever get drunk on vodka and Red Bulls – after all doesn't caffeine help to sober you up? NO! Why people drink loads of coffee to sober up is a mystery – all you end with is a more alert drunk! The liver can only process one unit of alcohol per hour and all the Red Bull and coffee in the world cannot speed up this process – in fact nothing can. This is because alcohol is a very highly toxic substance; in fact it is just as toxic as heroin. Let me reiterate this little known fact –

Alcohol is just as toxic as heroin

Despite this we have 'expert' doctors telling people that drinking some alcohol is better than not drinking it at all. Please bear in mind that the 'experts' once said exactly the same thing about smoking too. They will actually admit that alcohol can be dangerous, but then tell us that in small doses it can be good for people over the age of forty. Now how the hell did they come up with this? We hear this kind of claptrap all the time and yet we never really question it. Why? Because it has been put across by the 'experts' and, don't forget, part of our own addicted brain wants to believe it too. They claim that the health gains are for people over forty who 'may' be protected against heart disease. Yet 90 per cent of people over the age of 40 *do* drink alcohol and heart disease is *still* the number one killer in the UK. If alcohol helped fight against heart disease, as is the claim, then we should be the healthiest nation in the world and our incidences of heart disease would be almost nil. But we don't and it isn't.

The reality is that alcohol kills 40,000 people a year in the UK alone, that's 100 people a day. World-wide that figure is about 1 million people. It batters your liver, kidneys and pancreas; it dehydrates your body; destroys brain cells and can shrink your brain. It eats away your stomach lining, speeds up the ageing process, weakens eyesight and causes impotence, diabetes and obesity. It is a highly addictive drug that can and mostly does keep you a slave for life. It also causes unnecessary and often overwhelming cravings for carbs and sugars and, despite all of this, there is no warning on the label.

The authorities aren't about to make us more aware either – the UK government earns £10bn a year from alcohol. We as a nation spend £25bn on alcohol per year. To put that in perspective that's more than the annual spend on cloths, schools and hospitals. And the conditioning experts are allowed to spend over £200m blatantly advertising this highly dangerous, very addictive, often life- and soul-destroying drug – and just like the drug food advertisers they are certainly good at their job. The Budweiser boys are perhaps the best – with their colony of ants carrying bottles of Bud underground and partying, to their very funny Louie the frog 'bud-weis-er' ad and the most recent Watsssssssuuuuuup? ad campaign.

Just like any product which is selling and promoting a false need, the alcohol boys show images and situations over and over again to condition us into drinking their product at certain times. And they know if we do it enough, we will feel uncomfortable and incomplete when we don't do it. In fact just the thought of going 'on the wagon' for most people creates a feeling of fear and apprehension such is the hold this stuff appears to have over so many people. Yet before we started taking it we didn't need it. (I don't know about you but I can't remember coming home from a bad day at school and saying 'I've had a pig of a day mum, I could murder a pint'.) The need for the drug, like any drug food or drink, is created by the drug itself. The fact is that everything alcohol does, like all drug foods and drinks, is illusory. And if we thought about it, we would easily see that our 'reasons' for drinking this stuff just don't hold water.

We say that we love the taste of alcohol. But remember your first alcoholic drink – it tasted disgusting. Why? Because your body – the true expert – was saying 'You are feeding me poison. Could you please stop doing it.'

We say that alcohol helps us to relax, yet we have all been angry at times when drinking and have often, depending on the situation, felt uptight whilst drinking this apparent relaxant. When you see someone having a fight in a pub, do you think 'Quick, give them more alcohol they are clearly not relaxed enough'?

We all say it helps to give us courage, yet when we see someone of three foot nothing ready to take on Arnold Schwarzenegger after a few beers, we know that's not genuine courage – it's stupidity. Alcohol removes fear and as such prevents us from ever overcoming our genuine fears or apprehensions in certain situations. In order to be courageous we must overcome fear, in order to grow as a person we must overcome fear: if alcohol has taken away your fear there is none to overcome – this means you are not being courageous.

We say alcohol makes us happy, yet it is common knowledge that alcohol is a depressant and we have all experienced this effect at times. If you are feeling down, you can drink all the alcohol in the world, but you will still feel down. And look at all the trouble and violence on Friday and Saturday nights – the people causing it look happy don't they?

We say it helps us to socialize, yet when we see someone who is drunk during the day the last thing we want to do is socialize with them. It also makes you slur your words, makes you repeat the same point constantly and eventually makes you pass out – hardly sociable.

Everyone has this 'party' 'good time' image of alcohol – not only because that is the side which is constantly advertised, but also due to the fact that most of the situations where we drink alcohol are 'good', 'fun' and often 'party' occasions: Christmas, birthdays, meals out with friends, the weekend, watching the game, New Year's eve, on holiday etc. But aren't these all good times anyway? Didn't we enjoy these times before we started drinking without the need for alcohol? Of course we did. The problem is now we have 'bells'. We have such a link with alcohol and these situations that we believe these situations wouldn't be the same without the stuff.

It's time to realize that alcohol doesn't make a party – it just happens to be drunk at all parties because we have been conditioned to do it. I have been to plenty of parties where the alcohol was flowing and it was a good night, but I have also been to many parties where the alcohol was flowing, yet it was still a lousy party. Why? BECAUSE THE ALCOHOL DOESN'T MAKE THE PARTY, nor do the drug foods in bowls everywhere – it's the company, the banter, the interaction and the music which all determine whether the party is a success or not. The truth is that alcohol may not have made any parties, but it has certainly ruined many. Funny how the Bud boys don't advertise that. In fact the alcohol boys want to appear to be on your side – drink their beer and you can be as 'cool', as 'hip', as 'in' as us is their message. But I'd love to do a 'true' version of the advertising – can you imagine?

Watssssssuuuup?
'just chillin, in fact bloody freezing standing here half-cut waiting for a cab at 3am, all because I can't bring my car when consuming this drug drink – true'

Watssssssuuuup?
'just chillin here with a beer-gut the size of the Napa valley, watching the game – true'

Watssssssuuuup?
'just chillin, destroying brain-cells, shrinking my brain, not making head nor tail of the game – true'

Watssssssuuuup?
'just chillin, passed out, missing the game – true'

Watssssssuuuup?

'just chillin, watching the game on a hospital bed waiting for a liver transplant – true'

And it's obviously not just the Bud boys; the whole industry is at it. Does all this mean you can't have a glass of wine with a meal or a pint with your mates? NO, NO, NO. You can do whatever you like – the idea, remember, is to feel free and the *odd* glass of wine or pint is really not going to prevent you getting to Mauritius (so to speak). But at the same time I also want you to feel free *not* to drink. What a concept that is. Yes, go out for a non-drink and love the experience for the sake of it – you never know you just might get hooked.

'I had a great night last night – I must have, I can't remember a thing'

In case you are wondering, I personally quit alcohol over 6 years ago and really have no desire to start again. Why don't I drink? Well it's not because I *can't*, because I obviously *can* whenever I want to, it's also not because I'm a couple of haloes short of a sainthood, and it's not because I'm what society would describe as an alcoholic. It's because I can't see a reason to do it any more. I now go out more than ever before, I don't have to worry about driving my car or how I will feel for work the next day. I socialize more because I have the freedom not to drink alcohol. I can stay out later and I wake up earlier. I see much more of life and I have my Sundays back. Oh and I never, ever get a hangover! So why would I want to drink the stuff, what would it do for me? About as much as it would do for a child – nothing. It wouldn't make me happier (as it's a depressant) and it wouldn't help me to socialize (as it makes me slur my words and stupefies me – then it makes me pass out). It wouldn't help me to relax (as it overworks the organs and shatters the central nervous system). It certainly wouldn't improve my watching of 'the game' (the game doesn't change because you've got a beer in your hand). It wouldn't give me energy (as it takes tremendous nerve energy to deal with it) and even though it's a liquid, it wouldn't quench my thirst, only cause dehydration. It would also drain fluid from my brain, destroy brain cells, beat up every organ in my body and it would rob my accounts of insulin and calcium. Plus, which was always a biggy for me – it would cause fat to be stored in my body. So yes I can drink alcohol whenever I want to, it's just call me fuddy-duddy – I just don't want to spend my one and only life exercising constant control, week in week out, over a drug drink which gives no genuine benefits whatsoever.

The only time I have any kind of alcoholic drink is for ritual purposes and nothing else. If someone's cracking open a bottle of bubbly to clebrate a special occasion, even though I may not agree with the conditioning around Champagne, I'll take a glass, say cheers, clink my glass with others, take a swig and go back to my normal drink. The hook would only occur if I thought that a particular occasion wouldn't be the same without actually *drinking* a certain amount of alcohol.

Clearly there are people who can and do have the 'odd' drink and it is their *genuine* choice, but the reality is that is rare. For *most* people the thought of having any kind of social gathering and not drinking would create tremendous fear within them and fear of that kind = HOOKED!

Clearly it's your choice and you may well not be hooked and be perfectly happy to just have a couple of glasses of wine with your restaurant meal, but be aware. What we think is our genuine choice is far from it. Our actual decision to take this drug drink is due to being under the influence. Most people think they are 'under the influence' when they actually imbibe alcohol. The truth is that the only reason why people even want to drink this stuff is because they are *already* under the influence. Under the influence of advertising, under the influence of misinformation, under the influence of others, under the influence of social pressure, and under the influence of the illusion created by the drug itself – which all adds up to the 'drunk blind' syndrome.

And as you can now see we have not only been eating all kinds of junk and drug foods blindly, but drinking all kinds of diet, soft, energy, and alcoholic drinks blindly too. We need to see very clearly that *all* the drug foods and drinks I have mentioned thus far have several things in common:

They ultimately starve the body of life

They cause us to feel *more* hunger than is natural

They cause false hungers *on top* of a malnourished genuine one

They speed up the ageing process by overworking and battering every single organ in the body

They take tremendous nerve energy to breakdown, use and eliminate

They create food and drink hangovers of various degrees and jolt the central nervous system

They affect your mood

They are addictive

They help to cause eating disorders

They completely mess up your blood sugar levels –WHICH GOVERN YOUR HUNGER

They cause insulin to be secreted by an overworked pancreas

They use vital enzymes from your enzyme bank accounts

They dehydrate the body

They create voids and empty feelings

They contribute heavily to weight gain

They rob and pillage your body's bank accounts of its most vital asset – life force

And if that's not enough, they all cost us a fortune too. Yep, we even pay for the privilege of being mentally and physically abused by all this rubbish. Yes it's not just your body's bank accounts of enzymes, insulin and calcium that get robbed, what about your financial bank account? This is perhaps the only time you will be able to say that drug foods and drug drinks really do help you to lose...

24

Pounds and Pounds

But you won't lose those pounds off your waistline. Here are a couple of eye-openers regarding the money that is being wasted on empty foods and drinks that serve no purpose other than to 'sustain' your life and line the pockets of the pushers.

GROWING FAT ON THE PROFITS

As a nation the UK spends over £7m a day on drug-like fast foods from places like 'Kac-Donalds' – that's *seven million pounds a day*. That doesn't include what we spend on all the crisps, cakes, chocolates, biscuits, 'energy' bars, sugared sweets and the like. We now spend, wait for it, £4m on crisps per day. That's a mind-blowing 14 million bags a day in a nation of 60 million. We spend £4m a day on a product which is so de-natured that it eats holes in your blood vessels, loads your bloodstream with fat, clogs your veins and arteries, sends insulin levels soaring and makes not one jot of difference to a genuine hunger.

Chocolate is another shocker. Choc-heads will spend an absolute fortune on this highly addictive, fat-causing drug food – the average is about £8000 in a lifetime and that's only with a very conservative spending of £3 per week. I used to grab some kind of choc bar on my way to work every morning and one on the way back. That's easily more than £3 per week, especially if I add the extra choc bought on 'special' occasions – birthdays, parties, mood swings, friends coming round, the weekend etc.

Then, of course, we have the tremendous amount of money spent on drug drinks. And what a fortune we spend too. Just the alcohol alone will set you back over £100,000 in your lifetime. That is how much the *average* drinker will spend; for many the figure is a lot higher. Then you have the 'soft' and 'diet' drinks. In the UK alone we consume ten billion cans of fizzy drug drinks every year – five billion of which contain that lovely stuff aspartame. The cost of this works out to be in the region of £3–4bn a year. Then there's coffee and tea, the two most addictive drug drinks of them all. They're nice little earners for people like Starbucks, Costa Coffee, the PG Tips boys and, of course, the McDonald's gang. Yes, not content with just selling their own coffee in their 'restaurants', McDonald's have decided to give Starbucks and the like a run for their money with the launch of McCafes. They want a piece of the coffee bean pie and who can blame them. The average cup of coffee in Starbucks is in the region of two pounds. The average coffee addict has their fix seven days a week and if they only have one cup a day it works out at well over £36,000 in their lifetime. I wonder if that's why they called themselves star-*bucks*?

SUGAR RICH

And let's not forget that nasty white stuff you drop in your coffee. Sugar sells because it is a drug and on top of that it's one which tastes sweet, is described as a food and is given to people in various forms as a treat! And because it tastes sweet there is no need to even train yourself to like it in the first place – no wonder most of the western world is hooked on it. We consume over 100lb of the stuff *per person* each year, according to official figures. I believe it's more than that, especially when you take into account that just one can of cola contains 7 teaspoons of the stuff, ketchup is 27 per cent sugar and the stuff is in virtually all processed foods. Our slavery to this stuff keeps Messrs Tate & Lyle laughing all the way to the bank and leaves us, not only financially worse off, but physically poor too.

The financial costs of consuming these nightmare products doesn't simply end with the cost of the substances themselves, you also have to take into account the indirect costs of these drug foods and drinks. Okay so we could talk about the fact that the average alcohol drinker will spend £18,000 on taxis alone or that they spend a huge amount on cover-up drugs to try counteract their hangovers. But far more important is the cost to your health. The end result of continuing to eat and drink this rubbish is likely to be disease and ill-health. Now I do realize that our National Health Service is free, but I think it's fair to say that it's at breaking point and more and more people are going private. Even those who cannot afford to go private soon find the money when their life is at stake. I mean how much is your liver worth? How much for your kidneys? Your heart? These are times when people really wake up and realize that money means jack when it's a matter of life or death. The idea is to wake up **now**, do something **now** – not when you reach that stage. It's much, much easier to prevent than it is to cure.

And let's not forget these drug foods and drinks create fat and speed up the ageing process. So if you don't make the change after you've read this book, make sure you keep plenty of money aside for the tummy tuck, the liposuction, the face-lift and the expensive anti-ageing creams. And whilst we are talking about the money spent treating the symptoms, let's not forget that $32bn was spent on different diets, 'nutritious' shakes, slimming pills and other weight 'cures' in the US in the year 2000 alone. On top of that, $23bn was spent on work time lost due to drug and junk food related problems.

Isn't it mad? We spend an absolute fortune on drug foods and drinks that make us feel and look sluggish, fat, old, make our lives hell and cause depression – and we then spend another fortune treating the symptoms they cause. It wouldn't be so bad if we were spending all this money on stuff that made us happier, but it doesn't – in fact it does the opposite, that's why you are reading this book. So why do we do it? Are we all just a couple of dimes short of the full dollar? Or are we highly intelligent humans who have simply been robbed blind?

Even if these drug foods and drinks were free of charge I still wouldn't go near them. I was walking into a large supermarket the other day when a young lady came up to me with a tray of chocolates and some coffee. When I said no thanks she said, 'But they're free'. Free? In what way? There's no such thing as a free lunch remember. The first fix of any drug is always given free, but what do they end up costing you in the long run? And this stuff costs you physically, mentally, emotionally and financially. If they were giving out free heroin-laced foods and drinks would you have some just because they were free? I know we are not dealing with heroin, but we are dealing with drugs in one guise or another – so to me it's exactly the same. And would you put diesel in your petrol car just because they had a special offer on it?

'You can fool some of the people some of the time but not all of the people all of the time'

I don't know who said that but it appears they were wrong. The drug food and drug drink industries have been fooling us all for years. They really have been robbing us blind. We have been seemingly happily parting with our hard-earned cash because we have been blinded by the advertising and blinded by the illusory 'pleasure' of injecting a shot of this stuff into our bloodstream to end the low *it* caused. But we have also been blind to people's greed to make money out of us – no matter what the cost to our health. Until the blinkers are off we remain mentally trapped.

Breaking free of this trap doesn't take 'positive thinking' or willpower, it just takes an open mind to see the truth and then the courage to make the change.

'THE TRUTH WILL SET YOU FREE'

Whoever said this was bang on and for the unfortunate mice in the tale I am about to tell you, the truth is undoubtedly the only thing that will ever set them free from...

25

The Mouse Trap

A mouse is put in a cage and given natural food, water and a funnel containing pellets of a drug (which look like food).

There is a button to the side of the funnel which dispenses the drug pellets. In order for the mouse to get the drug it must hit this button with its nose. The natural food and water have always been in the cage, but the funnel containing the drug pellets is new. So out of curiosity the mouse hits the button and receives its first dose of the drug. The pellets have also been sweetened to cover up the foul taste of the drug, which the mouse would naturally be repelled by.

The drug pellets are designed to shatter the mouse's nervous system and at the same time create a false hunger and a false need. They are designed to play havoc with the natural, finely-tuned chemical balance of the body by rapidly raising the blood sugar levels of the mouse and then making its blood sugar fall rapidly. It's the instant rise and excessive fall which they are hoping will trick the mouse into *choosing* the pellet drugs over natural food – just like any other drug addict. To add to the fun the pellets are also designed to cause dehydration.

The scientist now removes the natural food and the mouse is left with just the pellets and the water. However, to make matters worse, the scientist replaces the water with a liquid drug. Once again, just like the pellets, this liquid drug has been heavily sweetened to trick the mouse into believing it is something good. This liquid drug is designed to do exactly the same things as the food pellets, except that it dehydrates the mouse even faster than the pellets.

Having no choice the mouse then hits the button, eats the drug pellets and drinks the liquid drug. Because of the nature of these substances, the mouse very soon starts to feel the effects of low blood sugar and dehydration (let's call this the withdrawal period). As soon as the mouse begins to feel these effects, what does it do? It hits the button for a pellet and drinks the liquid. Does the mouse now feel better and calmer than it did? Does ending this aggravation create a feeling of pleasure? The answers are yes and when this happens BOOM – it's hooked. Physically, of course, there is no hold and if the mouse just stopped hitting the button it would return to normal. But it won't stop because it's now mentally hooked on a false belief. I cannot repeat enough that it's the delusion which is the real hook. The mouse has no way of knowing what is really going on as the empty, insecure feelings are just the same as normal hunger and normal thirst and the minute he eats and drinks the substances those feelings subside – for a short while at least.

After the mouse has hit the button for a few days, the scientist puts the natural food and water back into the cage alongside the drug pellets and liquid drug. When the mouse feels hungry it recognizes the old natural food and takes some. But in no time at all it goes straight for the button again. After a while the mouse ignores the food and water altogether and chooses the pellets and liquid drugs. Why? Because the natural food and water will not *instantly* satisfy the mouse any more. The natural food will only satisfy a genuine hunger; it cannot instantly feed the false one. The false one needs to be starved out, in a similar way to withdrawal from a drug. The natural food was not designed to send sugar levels sky high in an instant, because sugar levels are not meant to fluctuate at this tremendous rate – it causes an imbalance in the body and mind.

The blood sugar levels would need *time* to level out for the body's natural balance to be restored. The mouse has no way of knowing this, it just feels an insecure hungry feeling and so is not about to wait for the feeling to go away naturally. As far as the mouse is concerned it won't just go away naturally, it's hunger and if you ignore it you die. That hunger needs to be satisfied, and the natural food just isn't *instantly* doing the job. All animals are designed not to ignore hunger, it is the single biggest driving force of our lives and our existence depends on ending it. When we feel hungry, we feel insecure and restless, it affects the way we think and our concentration. This is the body saying, 'forget everything you *think* is important – it's time to survive'. So when the mouse feels the crashing effect of such low levels of blood sugar it has an insecure feeling and it knows that feeling as hunger. If the drug food was taken away from the mouse when it felt these feelings, it would panic. You see, even though there might be plenty of natural food around, it won't give the mouse that instant 'hit' it's looking for. If it starts to feel apprehensive about this or starts to panic, what will happen? More empty, insecure feelings occur, identical to that of very low blood sugar or hunger. So the *overall* empty, insecure feeling is now huge and if the mouse still cannot find any instant 'hit' food or drink, even greater panic will set in and an even greater insecure feeling will occur – the majority of which is caused by *mental* panic.

So can you see that even though the mouse might be left with plenty of natural good food – which would help to rectify the fine chemical balance of its body and ultimately solve its problem – it would still go into a frenzy looking for some food that provided an *instant* hit (very similar to humans on a diet don't you think?). Can you also see that if the cage was the only place for the mouse to get the instant drug food you could leave it wide open and the mouse still wouldn't escape? If you think about it, it can't escape for it's no longer the cage that's keeping it there – it's the lack of truth. The mouse is mentally trapped by a simple physical confidence trick.

The truth is it would be too scared to leave the cage because just the thought of not being able to find more drug pellets would send it into a panic. Don't forget the mouse actually believes it cannot survive without the pellets – that is how much these things have affected its nervous system and way of thinking. Can you also see that even if the mouse gained weight, became tired and lethargic and even knew that it was indeed the drug pellets causing those particular problems, it still would *not* stop hitting the button. Why? Because it's still mentally trapped. The same insecure feelings would occur, the same panic and the same low blood sugar. And in that moment, when the sugar levels crash and the empty insecure feelings begin, the mouse would feel insecure and the mental desire to end the insecurities ASAP would be greater than a desire to be slim and healthy. The second after the insecure feelings go away, the mouse can think straight once again – but by then it's too late.

This, ladies and gentlemen, is the food trap and we are the mice. And white refined sugar, additives, chemicals and white carbs are the pellets.

In the actual experiment with the mouse, the drug affected the mouse so badly that it physically shook when it was in withdrawal. When it hit the button the shakes stopped. But in no time at all its nervous system began to be affected again. The shakes started again and what did the mouse do? Hit the button. Did the mouse feel better? Yes! But only better than it did a moment before and nowhere near as good as it felt before it pushed the button for the first time. Did it feel a sense of pleasure? Yes! But only the pleasure you would feel by putting down some heavy shopping – it's just the ending of the aggravation. The poor mouse has no idea that its central nervous system is slowly being destroyed by the drug; the drug is fooling the mouse into thinking that it is helping and there is a genuine pleasure in getting the instant hit. In other words the mouse is hitting the button blindly. The more the mouse shakes the more it hits the button, the more it hits the button the more it shakes. The mouse builds up such an immunity and tolerance to the drug that it still shakes even whilst it hits the button and is under the influence of the drug; just slightly less than a moment before. After a while the mouse just continues to hit the button, hit the button, hit the button – until it dies.

Believe it or not the scenario above is not something I made up – experiments like this are routinely carried out in drug tests (though I have changed certain parts to illustrate the point I want to make). I do not agree with this type of experiment, but it perfectly illustrates the principle of the food trap.

This is why there are hundreds of thousands of highly intelligent people who are constantly struggling not to eat certain foods. And this is despite the fact that they know these foods are bad for them and cause weight gain, lethargy and misery. The saying goes, 'what you don't know can't harm you' but it's not true in this case is it? What you don't know could eventually kill you.

If you look at the experiment it is exactly what I was doing when I was hooked on drug foods and drinks, and it is precisely what you and millions like you have been doing probably ever since you were first weaned. Once you hit the button a couple of times you really do become the mouse. The difference is that we had our first dose of refined sugar before we were old enough to think for ourselves. We are all meant to have a sweet tooth as fruit and nuts are our natural foods, so we were easily fooled on the taste front. And on top of that we have the advertisers actually encouraging us to hit their button and become their mouse. The more they get us to hit the button, the more money they make. And the fatter and more tired we become the more we think we need this stuff to keep us going (see the loop?).

FREE BLIND MICE

But, just like the mouse, we cannot see things for what they are whilst we are pushing the button – especially if we are surrounded by millions of people all doing the same thing. Drug foods and drinks *appear* to have the opposite effect to what they are really doing, so until someone points it out how the hell is anyone meant to see? These so-called foods were suppressing my nervous system so much that I believed in the end that I could not enjoy myself or live properly without them. Knowing what I know now, I wonder how I lived properly with them – oh that's right, I didn't. The insecurities and strong apprehensions I felt at just the thought of getting rid of this rubbish were all *caused* by the drug foods and drinks themselves. Just like the fears the mouse had were ultimately caused by the button. Now I am out of the cage it is easy to see that and now that I don't eat the drug pellets I don't have the insecurities or apprehensions. The reality is that there is nothing to fear by escaping from the trap and everything to fear by staying in it.

This book is about stepping outside yourself so that you can see what is really going on. If the mouse had the opportunity to see what it was actually doing, do you think that it would continue to hit the button? Do you think it would continue even if the drug pellets tasted sweet? Do you think it would continue if it knew that the insecure feelings would just go if only it *stopped* hitting the button? Would it continue if it knew that the button was the cause and not the cure? Do you honestly think for one second it would stick around if it was armed with the facts? Not in a million years.

The mouse never had a genuine choice, it was never *its* choice to hit the button, it was simply lured into a very clever trap, and ended up believing it was choosing to hit it. Exactly the same thing happened to me and exactly the same thing *is* happening to you and millions like you. No wonder we hate ourselves for eating this rubbish. We know it's bad for us, we know it's making us fat, and hate ourselves for doing it, but we've missed the main point – we never really understood *why* we were doing it. Everyone is so busy focusing on why we shouldn't eat rubbish (as if we don't know) they have failed to look at the simple chemical reactions created by the drug foods themselves; chemical reactions that cause false hungers and delude us all into believing we can't quit because we love these 'foods' too much.

Starve the false hungers from the body; get rid of the brainwashing from the mind; change your brand of food to the whole, natural versions and you are free – no more food problem ever. Wow! And it feels so bloody good I can tell you. To know that you will never be overweight again is a true feeling of total freedom. To feel light and have the raw energy to literally suck the juice from life is just the best feeling in the world. To wear what you want when you want to is a feeling I will never take for granted. To feel energetic, confident, slim and actually like the way you look and feel is like a new world. The best feeling of them all though is just not having to control what you eat: to be free from the constant battle with food. No more weighing food, no more weighing myself, no more feeling bloated, no more drug food hangovers. It's great to finally be free from always using a degree of willpower or discipline not to eat too much of certain foods; to be free from having to use self-control. No more discipline during the week, only to binge every weekend and 'diet' again every Monday. I used to think if I could manage my drug food intake during the week it proved I was in control. But in truth it proves the opposite – if you are having to exercise control you are not in control and you certainly aren't free.

The irony is that the only things keeping people in the food trap are their own thoughts and beliefs. The actual physical 'withdrawal' from these drug foods and drinks is hardly even noticeable, especially when you have some Juice Master fast food flowing through your bloodstream helping to restore the body's natural balance. Our thoughts and beliefs about certain foods and drinks have been influenced by years of brainwashing, conditioning and total bullshit from the food industries and their clever advertising friends. The excellent news is that the door to freedom is wide open and always has been; we have, in fact, been our own jailers – trapped by what we *believe* we get from these foods and drinks. The only reason people struggle when they go on a diet or try to change what they eat is because they strongly believe they are giving up a genuine pleasure that they think they can't be without. The fear is in the *thought* of 'missing out', the *belief* we are 'making a huge sacrifice'. Change the belief, see the truth and you realize there is nothing to fear. Once that happens you can break free – it really can be that easy.

But before you set off on any journey you need to be prepared, you need the correct directions and full understanding of what lies ahead to make certain that the change is permanent. Because of this I felt it wise to include a chapter on the sacrifices you will be making in the name of a slim, light and energy-driven body. Yes you read correctly, in the next chapter I have written in large bold letters a complete and comprehensive list of what you will be giving up.

26

What You Are
Giving Up

NOTHING!

... That's right – NOTHING! Oh, apart from feeling like crap, excess mounds of unwanted fat, a constant lack of energy, bloated feelings, indigestion, heartburn, the incredible frustration of not being able to wear what you want when you want to, the self-loathing, the guilt, the fear, the fat (did I mention the fat?), the lack of true courage and self-confidence, clogged-up veins and arteries, the undermining of your central nervous system, the battering of every single organ in your body, premature ageing, the stress on your body and mind, the beer gut (if you have one), the constant drug food and drug drink hangovers, hiding your body, the secret eating (I do know), feeling ashamed, the fat (well it was a big deal for me!), having to wear black, headache tablets, blood pressure pills, the mood swings, constantly weighing yourself, going on a diet every Monday, feelings of failure, and the fat, the fat, the fat, the fat – THE FAT. But what you will be 'giving up' most of all is...

The daily mental and physical slavery of being a drug food addict

You will be giving up just about the worst dis-*ease* you will ever suffer from – a progressive disease you probably didn't even realize you had, a disease which zaps your confidence and gradually pulls you lower and lower. You will be giving up being controlled and dictated to by drug foods and drinks. You will be giving up being subconsciously brainwashed every day by the junk and drug food industries. You will also very likely be giving up a good chance of becoming, or remaining, insulin dependent (diabetic), having a heart attack, a stroke or a seizure. And because what you put into your body affects every single organ and also the body's immune system, who knows what other horrors you will be 'missing out' on in your future life.

The fact is there is *nothing* to give up. Trying to weigh up the pros and cons of making the change is pretty easy in this case – THERE ARE NO CONS WHATSOEVER. What cons would the mouse have to face outside the cage? What would it be giving up if it just left? What sacrifice would it be making? None! All the sacrifices are made when you are in the trap. The Juice Master's mental and physical health recipe is so far from a diet it's a joke. Get it clear there is nothing to give up and no sacrifices to be made – that's the whole point of the book; to show you the confidence trick. We were all deluded because of some very clever advertising, (the 'bells'), a sweet taste and a trick involving our blood sugar levels and central nervous systems (the buttons).

You are not 'giving up' eating or living; on the contrary, you're going to start eating and living properly. You're not giving up the pleasure of eating good food – you will get more pleasure from *every* meal you eat from the time you make the change. You will be eating only when you feel a genuine physical hunger and you will be free as a bird to satisfy that feeling at will. Also be clear that you will not be making any sacrifices on the taste front either. I cannot emphasize enough that no matter how much you doubt it now, you will learn to enjoy the taste of anything you eat or drink on a regular basis. Your taste buds just need a bit of training that's all, as they've been out of shape for some time. Three weeks in the 'The Juice Master fresh food gym' is more than enough of a work-out and your taste muscles will be shaped for life. Remember, once you change your brand of food, you will not only love the taste but your new brand will do things the old one never could. It will satisfy and produce genuine hungers, it will feed every cell in your body, it will replenish your body's bank accounts oh yes, and it will free up some raw energy in your body which will help to flush out fat.

So apart from lethargy, excess weight, slavery, and all the other nightmare symptoms you get from being a drug food and drink addict – you really are giving up...

Nothing

If you can see that, if you have really opened your mind and understand that there is nothing to give up you will feel no sense of sacrifice whatsoever. And if you believe it now, why would you ever get uptight or miserable if you are *not* consuming this rubbish – what power on earth could ever convince you that you are missing out?

The truth will set you free and the truth is that you are not making any sacrifices. There is therefore no need to use your 'willpower' not to eat or drink this rubbish. Think about it, willpower only needs to be used when you are still fighting a desire to do what you still want to do. When you don't want to, there is no battle and you are free. And once you look at the simplicity of it, it becomes glaringly obvious why, not just physically but mentally, diets nearly always end up in failure. All they do is treat the *physical* symptoms of being *psychologically* hooked on the illusions the drug foods and drinks create. Unless you can see from the outside of the cage, diets are a no-win situation – especially if you are a strong-willed person. I used to be a tad confused with my will, as I was pretty strong-willed in most other aspects in my life, but so weak-willed when it came to certain foods and drinks. However, the opposite of what we've been led to believe is actually true. The *stronger* willed you are the *less* chance you have of suc-ceeding on a diet. You will begin to understand why as we look at the most common mental and physical recipe people follow in order to get a slim, healthy body – and you will see why it nearly always falls apart. It is of course...

27

The 'Diet' Recipe

A recipe for disaster

 I will now give you the traditional 'diet' recipe for solving your food, weight, energy and health problems – see if you can spot any flaws.

1 'Give up' the foods and drinks causing the problem.
2 Believe you are making a huge sacrifice and that your life will not be worth living.
3 Work yourself into a mental tantrum, like a child being told she will never be allowed to play until she's slim and healthy.
4 Get irritable with people around you (if you do this for long enough the people who told you to go on the diet will probably tell you to just go and eat).
5 Allow all of your waking thoughts to be dominated by thoughts about the foods and drinks you've 'given up'.
6 Feel sorry for yourself at all times (very important ingredient).
7 Stay in and feel constantly deprived. On no account go out and have fun.
8 Sit and wait for the desire for these foods and drinks to go away (using this recipe this should only last for the rest of your life).
9 Hate and envy all your friends who are allowed to eat and drink what you are being forced not to.

10 Weigh yourself every day to really feed the depression.

11 Eat when no one is looking, and when they are eat some cabbage soup.

12 Spend all the time you are on the diet moping around for something which you hope you'll be able to resist.

13 Starve your body so that you are also physically fighting against the most powerful instinct known to mankind – survival.

14 Eat less food than your body can function on so that your body begins to store *more* fat whilst it eats away at muscle tissue and slows *down* your metabolism.

Spot any flaws in the recipe?

If you followed all the ingredients that make up the diet recipe, do you think for one second you would feel happy about making the change? Do you think there's a chance in hell you could do this for the rest of your life? Can you see why 95 per cent of diets fail? I believe that the figure is 100 per cent, for how do you gauge success? By how much weight is lost? By how long they have kept it off for? By how much energy someone has? If someone is still using these ingredients to 'stay slim' or to 'stay healthy' then they have only been successful in using tremendous amounts of discipline, and continue to do so. But if you are still mentally craving certain foods and constantly using your discipline not to have them, you are not a success and you are still not totally free from the food trap.

I know not everyone reading this book is doing so to lose weight, but I have yet to find anyone who doesn't want more energy, better health and a strong immune system to help prevent 'normal' degenerative diseases. And those people who are already slim and trying to change what they eat still use the same mentality as those trying to lose weight; in other words they are still using the diet recipe, thus are also in the trap.

I personally used the diet recipe many, many times, always believing that the reason I could never hack it was simply down to the fact I had no willpower and was just weak-willed when it came to certain foods. But willpower had nothing to do with it; I just had no idea what was happening in my bloodstream and that I was addicted to drug foods. The term drug food has never been used so how is anyone meant to know it's the food that is the problem and not them.

It's not about how much willpower you have; in fact you know you are free when you no longer have to use willpower to control your intake of certain foods and drinks. For those of you who are convinced that quitting certain foods and drinks must require willpower, let me illustrate this point clearly. Imagine two people, one strong-willed and the other weak-willed, each with a chocolate bar in their hand ready to eat it. If you were to take the chocolate off them and tell them they can't have it, who do you think would kick up more of a fuss? Yes – the strong-willed one. Now imagine the same two people in a room with chocolate bars near them, but neither of them had any desire for them at all, they just didn't want them. What would happen if you were to come in and take the chocolate bars away? Which one is going to kick up more fuss? The answer is neither of them. Why? Because they don't want it, they have no desire for it, and they don't believe their lives would be enhanced by it. And if you really don't want something it becomes completely irrelevant whether you are weak-willed or strong-willed. But if you still believe certain foods retain a benefit and you use the diet recipe to try and do without them, then the stronger willed you are the *more* of a fuss you'll kick up.

The problem is every time you use this recipe, all you do is reinforce over and over again what you believe about these drug foods and drinks – that life with them is a hell of a lot better than life without. When you are on a diet you build these foods up in your mind to be something which they are just not. You believe they are beneficial to you in some way, therefore you feel deprived when you think about them. The more deprived you feel the more precious those foods become, the more precious they become, the more deprived you feel. It doesn't take long before you say, 'SOD IT'. Now try to imagine going through this mental tug of war whilst starving at the same time. No need to imagine, if you have been on any one of the common diets you have already experienced it. On most diets we are not just putting ourselves through a mental trauma, but also a physical one. Most diets involve nutrient and food deprivation – this is called starvation. When the body senses it is starving it starts storing what?

FAT. Whilst you are starving, your body begins to eat your muscle tissue, leaving the fat till last for energy. You are now starving your body of food and nutrients to an even greater degree than normal and it's not even getting enough bulk to sustain a reasonable quality of life. Your sugar levels remain at a lower level than is comfortable, thus creating a knock-on effect in the mind which is now screaming to feel satisfied. No wonder you get ratty, irritable and say 'sod it'. Are you happy when you have first 'given in' to your own mental and physical tantrum? YES, of course. You feel better because you've just been through mental torture and hell and, depending on the diet, you have been physically starving yourself at the same time. So we are bound to feel an immediate sense of total relief when we stop the mental tantrum and feed the body.

On top of that, when we are using the ridiculous diet recipe we avoid going out where possible, and if we do brave the outside world we're constantly looking at all the food other people are 'allowed' to eat – so either way it's hell. We constantly feel deprived, so we strongly believe we are making huge sacrifices. And on a diet we go through this mental tug of war for hours, days, weeks, or if you are some kind of truly amazing human (or masochist), months or even years. So when we say 'Oh sod this for a game of soldiers' and decide to bring the madness to an end – WE ARE BOUND TO FEEL BETTER. But that is only because we have put ourselves through mental hell in the first place: once again the satisfaction and pleasure we feel is in the ending of a massive low.

When a baby is crying it's enough to make you pull your hair out and when they fall asleep it's total bliss. But the pleasure you experience is just the ending of the low. I mean you wouldn't deliberately start a baby crying just to feel the relief when it finally shuts up would you? (if you answered yes, you really are in need of a different kind of therapy).

The problem is when we say decide to 'give in', we don't realize that the relief and pleasure we then get from eating the foods we were craving is just the ending of a massive mental and physical aggravation which we have caused in the first place. So the pleasure this gives simply confirms in your mind that you are miserable, boring, unsociable and ratty individual *without* those types of food and much happier with them. This only adds to the ingrained belief that these foods are very precious and pleasurable, and help your mood. We deduce from all of this that we are indeed happier because of these drug foods and drinks. Yet the truth is we are happier *because* we have stopped a mental tantrum, which we and only we were causing.

It wouldn't be so bad if the battle came to an end when we did decide to 'give in', but what caused the mental battle in the first place? Yes indeedy – the very foods themselves. We are using the foods which caused the battle to begin with as a tool to try and end it. This is why the battle *doesn't* come to an end by simply going back to the old ways. By having these foods again we may be happier than we were on the diet, but only for a very short time. In fact usually only half way through the piece of drug food we ate, because we soon realize what we have done and start to feel like a weak-willed failure once more and delude ourselves that this 'one off' won't hurt and all will be okay. But too late – the drug food parasites have reared their ugly heads and you have just seemingly had confirmation that you were missing out. The dripping tap has well and truly started and now you are using each mental ingredient of the diet recipe magnified 1000 per cent in your head. The battle has not come to any kind of an end with that 'sod it', it's just become a whole lot tougher.

You then spend the next couple of days or weeks deluding yourself that you are still on 'it' and yet are seemingly blind to all the secret eating you are now doing. After all, it's one thing for you to know you have failed, it's another to tell the world. So it's salad in front of your friends and pig-out when you're by yourself! After you have had enough of hiding the fact that you are now eating this rubbish again, you then let everyone know by blaming the diet itself or your genes (always a good one). You say you have been on 'it' for much, much longer than you actually were, and as the people around you only actually saw you eating salad, they believe you. You then start to eat the same way as you did before you went on the diet, only now you binge slightly more, subconsciously trying to make up for all that lost time. After a couple of months of 'living' like this, with all the physical side effects that go along with the intake of drug and junk foods, you realize you really can't live like this and so try and solve the problem once more by going on a what? Um – see the problem? But nothing has changed; no matter which 'diet' you now choose, you are still going to have a battle because the problem is mental not physical. So we end up going nuts spending our lives on a semi-permanent diet, constantly trying to control our intake of foods and drinks which are controlling us, whilst still keeping all the physical symptoms of being a drug food addict.

The 'diet recipe' only removes the foods and drinks causing the problem – in fact many diets don't even do that – but you are still left with the brainwashing. The food problem is in reality 95 per cent mental and only 5 per cent physical. If you only remove the physical you are still left with a very, very big problem. You are still left with the very strong belief that you are missing out. You are still left with the belief that you cannot enjoy or cope with your life in the same way without these foods and drinks. In other words you still have the problem.

There are many people who have quit drug and junk foods, but still have a problem with them. If they've quit but six months down the line are still craving all those drug and junk foods, using their control not to have them, then these people still have a food problem – even though they don't actually eat these foods. Even if these people do get slim, they still have a food problem and because of this the chances of them *staying* that way are not good.

This is why 'Fat Camps' and health breaks rarely work. People pay huge sums of money to be locked in some building in the desperate hope that when they are 'released' they will be slim. But the cause of the problem isn't tackled at all – only the symptoms. They are *still* using the diet recipe when they're in these places, which means as soon as they're 'released' they will immediately reward themselves for being 'good'. And what do they reward themselves with? Exactly!

According to conventional wisdom, then the choice seems to be one of two options. Either eat the junk and drug foods and suffer the daily mental and physical consequences or try to stop consuming them using the 'diet recipe' and suffer the daily consequences of that nightmare. Either way you still suffer and you still have a food problem.

There is of course one other option that no one seems to have thought of – see the foods for mind-controlling, body-destroying substances that they really are and jump for joy to be finally free *not* to have to eat them.

There are many 'food gurus' who have made millions out of helping people who are overweight, but are far from ecstatic about being free themselves. The main reason for this is they are not free. Many, like Rosemary Conley, might be slim but they still believe they are making many sacrifices when it comes to certain foods and drinks; they just believe that the sacrifices are worth it. But as the previous chapter illustrated, all the sacrifices are made when you are having to eat this rubbish day in day out, not when you're not. All the sacrifices are made when you suffer the mental and physical problems these so-called foods create. These people should be over the moon to be free from the fat, the lethargy, and the slavery to these types of food. But many of them are still *mental* slaves to these foods, even though they might be physically okay now, they just use their discipline to control them to a certain degree.

As far as Rosemary Conley, the big weight loss clubs and virtually all the 'food' gurus are concerned it's all about exercising control. Sarah Ferguson, the duchess of York and one of the 'faces' of Weight Watchers, said of the overweight people featured on a TV programme on obesity, ' It will be a life-long battle for all of them'. And the sad thing is it will be unless they see the truth – if they see the truth they can be free. Do you want to exercise control for the rest of your life or do you want to be free?

Instead of achieving mental and physical freedom from these drug foods and drinks most of us simply 'cut down' on the amount of the *same* food we were eating in the first place – smaller portions and weighing scales. The calorie counting madness that has been the heart of the diet industry for decades is all about counting and cutting down. The same goes for 'points' and 'sins'. But when you 'cut down' on these foods, not only can you never achieve your goal of total mental and physical freedom, but you once again make these foods and drinks appear *more* precious than before – making the 'hook' even stronger. After all, the longer you hear a baby crying the more pleasure you feel when it finally stops!

There are people out there that can tell you exactly how many calories are in virtually every food – and I mean to the exact number! During the obsessive counting calorie days, which to be fair are far from over, some people even worked out that a cheese sandwich had exactly the same amount of calories as semen! Then you have slimming clubs not only doing their completely pointless counting the points stuff, but also the food diary nonsense. But how is writing down everything which passes your lips this meant to help? Any dieter worth their salt will know that if you eat anything while you are standing, or from someone else's plate, or you just take little bites of something every now and then, you won't put it in your diary because in any of these situations IT DOESN'T COUNT! And anyway, who the hell has got the time to actually list everything they eat and drink? More importantly why on earth should we want to?

It seems slightly mad that as intelligent human beings we think that if we do somehow manage to cut down on the junk, keep a food diary, weigh our portions of food correctly, check what time we are allowed some more food, see how many 'points' or 'sins' we've got left for the day etc. etc. that it proves we are in full control of our food. But if you think about it, the opposite is true. If you have to do any of this it proves you are far from in control, in fact it proves you are being controlled by the very things you believe you are in control of. Remember –

**If you are having to exercise control over anything,
then that something must be controlling you**

The idea is to stop trying to control and just free yourself both mentally and physically – then you become truly in control. In reality people like Rosemary Conley, and most people on a diet, are con-stantly moping around for certain drug-like foods and drinks which they hope they won't have. Can you imagine doing that? Once again, there's no need to imagine it as we have all been guilty of making the whole process of changing what we eat very hard for ourselves by doing precisely that.

WE CONSTANTLY MOPE AROUND FOR CERTAIN FOODS AND DRINKS WHICH WE HOPE WE WON'T HAVE

Isn't that just a touch mad? A tad nutty? Isn't it bonkers to spend your life moping around for certain things which you hope you won't have? And this is the main reason why we all think it's difficult to get rid of certain foods and drinks from our lives. Yet if we just stopped the moping and the self-imposed feelings of deprivation and actually felt good about the fact we now have a genuine choice and are totally free *not* to consume the crap any more, we just might find the whole process not only easy but enjoyable.

We would also find it a hell of a lot easier if we didn't tell ourselves over and over again that we can't have certain foods or drinks when in reality we can do what the hell we like. I used to have chocolate most days, but there would be times when I just didn't have any for many days. Did it bother me? No! Was I using willpower in the time I had no desire for it? No! Did I suffer withdrawal? No! And many of you reading this book will have had many occasions where you have gone for days without having certain foods and drinks and yet it hasn't bothered you in the slightest. But the very second you tell yourself you *CAN'T* have these things any more, boom! – you experience the 'forbidden fruit' syndrome. When this happens the 'forbidden' foods and drinks become a thousand times more precious than they were before you told yourself you couldn't have them. The result? You immediately feel miserable and deprived, even if you would normally find it easy to abstain for a few days.

Get it very clear in your mind that when you get rid of the drug-like foods and drinks from your life, you CAN consume them whenever you wish, just as I can whenever I wish. I just *don't* wish. You CAN, after all, take heroin whenever you wish; nobody in the world is stopping you, so why don't you? Because you don't wish to. I am not your teacher or parent, you CAN do whatever you want after you read this book – the choice is yours. But please remember you will no longer have a choice if you *do* consume all these drug-like foods and drinks. Drug addiction of any kind takes away the freedom of genuine choice. It must be crystal clear that we are not talking about a habit or a genuine pleasure or even genuine food – it is *drug*-food addiction, nothing less.

Bear in mind though that the addiction is virtually all psychological. If you tell yourself that you can't then you will feel deprived and miserable. What we should be saying is, 'I *can* have these foods and drinks, but what on earth would be the point, what would they do for me?' The answer to that question is crystal clear – NOTHING. There is just no point in eating or drinking these nightmare substances, other than in emergency situations.

Just saying the word 'can't' or actually believing that you *can't* would be the only thing that could make it remotely difficult for you to quit the drug foods. I have a couple of great acronyms for the word can't –

Constant And Never-ending Torture
and
Constant And Never-ending Tantrum

That is exactly what we put ourselves through when we keep telling ourselves we *can't* – constant and never-ending torture. Look at Rosemary Conley: judging by the article I read she is, at certain times, suffering from the CAN'T syndrome. She wrote the incredibly successful *Hip and Thigh Diet* donkeys years ago, which would strongly suggest she is doing the 'never-ending torture' bit quite successfully. But why put yourself through a completely unnecessary mental torture?

Once you are out of the cage you *can* go back in whenever you want. You *can* suffer the daily nightmare of being dependent on drug foods that are doing nothing for you. You *can* remain fat, lethargic and hooked, but if you now understand what is going on, why on earth would you ever want to? The point is that you *can* have whatever you want whenever you want – not that you *can't*. What you say to yourself determines how you feel about any situation. By understanding at any time that you always can but that there is no point to it, you instantly remove the T, which is where the torture lies. All we need to do is shift from the diet mentality, which is –

'I want but I *can't* have'

to the correct way of thinking –

'I *can*, but I don't want to have'

Or more accurately:

I can, but I don't *need* to, or *want* to – I'm free

Many of my friends and family still say, 'Oh I forgot you can't have that can you' or 'Let's look on the menu to see what you can have'. What they fail to realize is that I can have whatever I like – often they are the ones being controlled by their eating habits, not me.

We have all at some point in our lives suffered from the 'can't' syndrome. It's the syndrome everyone experiences when they're quitting smoking or alcohol or are on a diet. The mad thing is it's self-inflicted and so easily remedied. Did being told 'you can't' stop Adam from picking an apple from the tree? Did being told he would die if he did, make any difference? NO. Why? Because…

C.A.N.T. overrides death

And there are many people who, at this moment, are being told to either diet or die. Many, unfortunately, will die: not because they are weak-willed, but because they are caught in a very clever trap and are under the illusion that they will be missing out if they quit the rubbish and start to eat and drink healthily.

As soon as Adam told himself he couldn't have that apple, he was doomed. Adam simply fell victim to the can't syndrome. Tell yourself you can't and you will want whatever it is you think you can't have a thousand times more. Understand you can – that nothing is preventing you but that there is just no point in having it, that you don't actually want to – and you won't struggle. It isn't hard and for the first time ever you'll feel free.

I cannot emphasize enough that the reason why people find it difficult to quit the kinds of foods and drinks that are causing them so many problems has got *nothing* to do with their genetic make-up, character, or personality: it is simply down to a feeling of *mental* deprivation – a mental moping caused by the belief that they are missing out on some kind of genuine pleasure. They feel mentally upset because society's attitude has perpetuated the belief that if you don't eat and drink these drug-like substances, *you* are the one making the sacrifices (and, of course, this is reinforced by the illusory effects of the drug foods themselves). You believe that these substances are affecting *your* life, but most people can seemingly eat and drink this stuff without the same problems. This is simply not true – the need itself, the actual desire to consume these drug foods and drinks is the problem. Putting these substances into your body is the problem. The need to try and exercise constant control is the problem. And that's without the physical side-effects of fat, tiredness and lethargy.

GOING GREEN WITH ENVY

Get it clear, *everyone* who feels the need to consume this rubbish on a regular basis is in the cage and *has* the problem. Whether they actually admit it or not is irrelevant as we need to bear in mind that *all* drug addicts lie – including drug food addicts. So the last thing we should be doing is envying people who still remain in the food trap; instead we should feel sorry for them. If you saw your best friend in the cage hitting the button over and over again would you envy them? Would you feel as though you were missing out? Or would you attempt as best you could to explain exactly what they are doing so they too could be free? The point is simple – don't envy these people, why not change what you have always done and actually start to *pity* them instead and feel euphoric about the fact that at least you are free?

No wonder we all believe it's hard to lose weight, gain health and have physical and mental vibrancy – we have all been going about it back to front. People *start* their attempt to get a slim, energy-driven body believing that it will be very difficult. They dread it and who can really blame them? They strongly believe they will be making huge sacrifices; that it will be very, very hard; that their life will change for the worse; that they *can't* have these foods any more; that they are going to feel constantly deprived and miserable; that they are going to envy everyone they see; and, if they do manage to reach their ideal health and weight, in order to stay that way they will have to use 'control' and 'willpower' for the rest of their lives. It sounds like living hell and no doubt if you have tried to change what you eat in the wrong way you'll have realized it is a living hell.

But as I can personally testify, if you do it right, then you can approach the change feeling not just positive but excited and elated. We have been so brainwashed into believing that a problem with food is a lifetime battle – that it is strange not to consume chemical concoctions masquerading as food – that we all begin our attempt to quit this muck by feeling sorry for ourselves, as if *we* have just made a massive sacrifice. This is instead of feeling liberated and elated at the knowledge that we have just freed ourselves from one of the worst forms of slavery from which we will ever suffer; that we have just stopped what is a progressive disease in its tracks. When you get rid of these foods from your life and step outside the cage, mentally and physically, it is the end of a disease and should be a wonderful feeling. But people using the diet recipe never get that wonderful feeling of freedom.

When people are on a diet they wind themselves up into a mental tantrum. The theory is that if you can suffer the tantrum for long enough the cravings for certain foods will eventually go and you will reach the stage where you can tell the world, 'Have you heard the news? I don't need to eat that rubbish any more – I'm free'. Let me ask you a question: at what stage did Nelson Mandela *realize* that he was free from his captors? At what point was he free never to return ever again? Was it a year after he was released? A month? A week? A day? Or was it the very second he was released? Do you ever think he gets a craving to go back in? Of course not – he's over the moon to be free.

But at what point can the ex-drug food and drink addict say, 'Have you heard the news? I've done it. I'm FREE: I'm free *not* to consume this rubbish any more. Isn't it wonderful?' At what point in their lives can they become elated that they are free? At what point will the 'craving' go? At what point can they be over the moon to be free? The answer is *never*, not while they believe that they are still missing out.

The problem is that the attitude of society, the brainwashing and the years upon years of advertising all combine to give you the impression that if you are *not* eating fat-causing, life-destroying foods that you have indeed made a genuine sacrifice; that you will be the one who is missing out, that you will become boring and unsociable. So when people quit these nightmare foods and drinks they don't start by celebrating the fact they are free from products that have been mentally and physically abusing them, but rather with a feeling of complete despondency wondering *when*, not if, they will fail.

The big trauma that the 'dieter' goes through when they stop eating certain foods and drinks is not caused by the withdrawal of the drug-like foods leaving their body, or by anything in their genes, but by a feeling of MENTAL DEPRIVATION. And people only continue to feel deprived because they don't know the full nature of the subtle and sinister food trap. You, on the other hand, now do. Which would make it even more ridiculous for you to continue pining for this rubbish *after* you break free from it. It would be the same as Nelson Mandela pining for prison. Can Nelson go back to prison? Yes of course, but do you think he wants to? Of course not. What about if all his friends were in there? Do you think he would be jealous or envious of them? Or would he be over the moon that he is free and do everything in his power to help his friends get out?

You now know all the lies and rubbish we have been subjected to since birth about certain foods and drinks, which means you have the unique opportunity to free yourself from drug foods and be happy about it. And now that you do have an understanding of drug foods, drug drinks, the bullshit advertising and the misleading labels you are finally in a position to deal successfully with the *physical* symptoms of being a *mental* victim of the food trap. And if you are anything like I was, you probably have a lot of physical symptoms from a lifetime of consuming the wrong kinds of foods and drinks.

In all likelihood you've been left with excess fat stored around many parts of your body; battered organs; elevated sugar levels; a dodgy ticker; a very depleted enzyme bank account; a clogged colon; waste matter circulating in your bloodstream, veins and arteries; and possibly arthritis, asthma, or diabetes. You will also probably have sticky blood cells and very low energy levels. In fact, we have clogged our systems so much over the years that there is a good chance that your colon has a build up of waste matter which has gradually hardened and stuck to its walls over the years, reducing what is normally a 6cm wide tunnel to one as small as just a few millimetres. Or, in other words, it's like trying to shove a watermelon through a polo mint! We are now, and it's official –

The most constipated nation in the world with 20,000 new cases of bowel cancer every year

Your colon is constipated, your arteries are constipated, your blood is constipated, your veins are constipated or, as one of my clients so elegantly put it, 'No wonder we feel like shit a lot of the time, it's because we're full of it' – well quite! Let's face facts: the body needs some physical help.

Now wouldn't it be incredible if there were a pill which could deal with the physical symptoms of being a victim of the food trap? A pill we could take every morning which would flush the leftover waste matter from our body, give us loads of energy and at the same time help repair damage to organs and tissue in the body? A pill which had been proven beyond doubt to have no adverse side-effects whatsoever and one which helped to fight and prevent disease. WOW – what if, can you imagine?

Well the exciting news is there really is no need to imagine – such a pill really does exist. It is time to unveil the most amazing health and weight loss discovery ever – ladies and gentlemen I give you...

28

The Ultimate Fat-busting Health Pill

 Imagine receiving a call from your doctor about news of an amazing breakthrough in health and weight loss science. In fact, it is the biggest breakthrough they have ever had. Nothing whatsoever has ever come close to the health-giving, energizing and fat-shifting powers of what he is describing as 'the ultimate fat-busting health pill'. He says that if you take the pill at certain times and at the correct dose you are guaranteed to get a slim, healthy and energy-driven body – yes, he said, *guaranteed*. He also makes it quite clear there are no adverse side effects and that he also has no vested interest in the pill at all. His only interest is to genuinely help you as he knows this amazing breakthrough will change every single aspect of your life.

He then sets out the guidelines for taking the pill. In order for this amazing pill to be *most* effective, it should be taken on an empty stomach. He suggests first thing in the morning, as you can be almost guaranteed that your stomach will be empty then. Now so far would this pose any problem to you? Would you take the pill under these conditions? Who wouldn't, hardly a penance now is it? However, he then says that if you really want it to work you should take the pill and *nothing* but the pill until about 12–2pm. Would this pose any problems? Well I, for one, wouldn't be doing cartwheels at the thought of eating just a pill for breakfast! However, the doc then goes on to explain that these little beauties don't look like, nor are like, any other pill on the planet.

UN-PILL-IEVABLE!

Each pill is made up of at least 80 per cent organic water. Some come with a tough outer layer – you simply take this off and eat what's underneath. Others come with a thin protective layer and you can just eat the whole lot. Wow – pretty amazing stuff! And before you start thinking there's got to be a catch, let me assure you there isn't: these pills have been specially designed to feed every single cell in your body. They contain every single vitamin and mineral known to mankind and many more that have yet to be discovered. They also contain enough calcium and essential fats to keep you fit, strong and healthy.

The design is even more remarkable as the high water content of the pills helps to transport all the goodness directly where the body needs it and helps to flush out the waste. The pills also require little or no digestion as they come with their very own digestive enzymes and have more or less been pre-digested. They take no nerve energy from the body, all they do is give you loads of the stuff. Because no digestion is needed for breakdown and disposal of the pills, energy is freed up to be used for repairing damaged tissues and organs, and to shift stores of fat. The pills are designed to totally satisfy a *genuine* hunger, leaving you feeling satisfied for longer and, due to the incredible amount of water they contain, they also are designed to meet the body's requirement for fluid. The specially-designed pills also contain enzymes which help with the break down and disposal of waste matter (i.e. excess fat). They are also specially formulated to help build an incredibly strong immune system, which helps to protect against every disease known to mankind. They not only give you genuine energy boosts without robbing your body's insulin bank account, but they have been designed to keep your sugar levels balanced. They help to strengthen bones and teeth, and improve breathing. They are designed to feed the body *and* the mind. They also improve concentration and mental agility, and have the amazing ability to enable you to sleep like a baby. WOW! WOW! and WOW again!

Sounds too good to be true? Well, before you get too excited, as with any pill you must be prepared for the inevitable side effects.

THE SIDE EFFECTS

Continued use of the pills has indeed brought with it many side effects. They have been heavily linked to an obscene amount of energy, shiny hair, strong teeth, hard nails and beautiful glowing skin. Another major side effect is having to cope with a slim body for the rest of your life and the improved sex life which comes along with more energy, feeling light and looking and feeling more attractive (oh no!). You may also find you have to throw out a lot of clothes as they will become too *big*. An unprecedented growth in courage, confidence and self-respect has also been attributed to these pills. There is a strong possibility you may also suffer the side effect of an improved cash-flow due to being more efficient both physically and mentally at whatever it is you do. Overall the warning on the label is crystal clear:

Be careful. This product will seriously improve every single area of your life

And that's not all – the pills come in hundreds of mouthwatering flavours, and all of them have an unbelievably sweet taste. That's right, they even taste good. And when I say taste good, I mean really good. Not just 'Oh we can put up with the taste for the sake of our health' type of good – I am talking deliciously divine. Here are just a few of the amazing flavours they come in: peach, pineapple, banana, mango, paw paw, orange, apricot, avocado, tomato, blackberry, strawberry, blueberry, melon, nectarine, kiwi, apple, tangerine, cherry, grapefruit, lemon, lime, grape, cucumber, sweet pepper, and hundreds more.

What's more, you don't need a prescription for these life-changing pills, because there are no adverse side effects. The pills are suitable for all ages, and can even be taken by pregnant women. You can also buy them virtually any where you go. Not only that but they are cheap too. In fact, given the money you save on drug foods, these hunger-satisfying, fat-busting health pills will save you a small fortune. Luckily for us the ingenious scientist who invented this amazing set of pills did so *not* in order to make millions, but simply for the well-being of others (how unique). This is why it is possible to get the pills for as little as 5p each – sometimes even cheaper. In fact, if you have your own garden you can even grow the pills yourself for free.

Having weighed up the pros and cons would you be interested in these amazing set of pills? ARE YOU KIDDING – WHO WOULDN'T? Would you be happy and excited to take them? Of course. How much willpower would you need in order to start taking them? None. In fact, having heard about the amazing benefits, you would only need willpower if you had to *restrict* your intake of them! But wait there's more, just when you thought it couldn't get better, these pills also contain tons of digestive enzymes which help to break down any of the non-natural foods you *do* eat and help to dispose of the waste they produce – simply amazing.

PIP-SQUEAKS

There are so many highly intelligent scientists out there in labs right now wasting their valuable time trying to find the ultimate fat-busting health pill. Well guess what guys and gals – IT ALREADY EXISTS. It fact, it has existed since the dawn of time. Yes indeed, as you've undoubtedly guessed, as simple as it sounds, fresh ripe sweet delicious *fruit* is indeed the ultimate fat-busting health pill. But then you hardly need to be Inspector Clouseau to work it out once it's been explained properly do you? Yet for some reason it has never been advertised for what it is and what it does, although I read that is all to change – thank God. Yes, finally schools will be giving fresh fruit to pupils. In addition, an advertising scheme is to be tested that will encourage children to choose fruit for themselves by making it 'hip and trendy'. I said advertising works and how's this for evidence? Children were shown videos featuring fruit- and vegetable-loving 'dudes'. They were told if they too eat these foods, they can join the struggle to defeat the evil General Junk and his Junk Punks. The results were mind-blowing.

Among children who watched the video, which contained snappy phrases and catchy songs, the consumption of fruit and veg increased FOUR-FOLD. That's simply amazing and in terms of the next generation's health it's a good start.

Fruit is the very food which we are, without doubt, biologically adapted to eat over any other food. No other food even comes close to the health-giving and cleansing properties of fresh ripe fruit. Scientists and food 'experts' can bang on as much as they like about what we should or should not be eating, and continue trying to create pills for health and weight loss, but no one can dispute that humans have the digestive tract of a primarily fruit-eating primate and the ultimate fat pill has *already* been invented – sorry guys and gals! Become your own scientist and see, feel and live the results.

There is no question that if you take the fat-busting health pill in its natural state at the times and in the amounts I will specify – and you follow my advice on meals for lunch and dinner – you will get slim and healthy. A bold statement to make, but it's a fact.

'AN APPLE A DAY KEEPS THE DOCTOR AWAY – AND THE LIPO SURGEON TOO'

(with a few apricots, oranges, bananas, avocados and nuts thrown in)

Hippocrates, the so-called 'father of medicine', knew only too well the power of fruit and veg. 'Let food be thy medicine' was his catchphrase and he was certainly right. If you are fat, you are ill; if you are tired all the time, you are ill; if you have arthritis, you are ill. If you feel like crap all of the time, you are ill. Mounds of fat are your body's way of telling you it is at dis-ease with itself: in other words, it has a disease and you are ill. And the only thing physically keeping all that fat there is a lack of nutrients and available energy. The body spends so much time trying to digest the rubbish we put in it that it simply doesn't have the time or energy to shift the excess fat, repair damaged organs, or to give us some mental or physical energy when we need it. If we just learn how to 'free up' energy in the body and provide it with a high-powered nutrient workforce, then the actual physical side of getting a slim, energy-driven body is very, very easy. The body just needs some help – and *fast, nutrient-packed food* is what it's crying out for.

I will repeat this point once more as I want you to really get this – the human body was specifically designed with *fast food* in mind, and once again I don't mean burgers and fries. I mean foods that are *fast* to digest, *fast* for the body to assimilate and *fast* for the body to eliminate. I mean real, genuine fast food: foods that will quickly inject nutrients into every cell in your body, giving it a brand new workforce that is specifically designed to clear out excess fat and wastes; foods that contain antioxidants which help to build a defence against cancer and other diseases; foods that contain massive amounts of what our body thrives on and cannot do without – water. This amazing group of foods not only taste incredible, but also help to replenish your already depleted enzyme and life bank accounts. And they don't leave you feeling bloated and guilty, but instead lift your spirits and keep you looking and feeling fantastic. Yep you can't beat them.

FRUIT AND VEG – THE DYNAMIC DUO

Even when I say it, it sounds too simple. But, yes, fruit and water-rich, easily-digestible veg are indeed nature's ultimate fast foods and the benefits of eating this amazing stuff every day last a lifetime.
I cannot say enough about fruit and veg – they are truly amazing.
Fruit and veg are about the only genuine foodstuffs that you could stick the following label on and in no way would it be misleading the public:

- No artificial colouring
- No preservatives
- No additives
- No added sugar
- No added salt
- No E numbers
- 99.9 per cent fat free

- 🍓 Non dairy
- 🍓 Water rich
- 🍓 Calcium enriched
- 🍓 Vitamin and mineral enriched
- 🍓 Suitable for old, young and can even be taken when pregnant
- 🍓 Totally natural
- 🍓 Pure goodness

But because they are natural, in the *genuine* sense of the word, they don't even need a label. It is super-fast, super-rich, super-charged nutrition. Fruit takes little or no digestion and so leaves the stomach very quickly, usually after about half an hour. It then goes straight to the intestines where the nutrients can be absorbed. It requires no washing up, tastes wonderful, looks amazing, satisfies a *genuine* hunger, is cheap compared to most other things, and the high water content helps to transport the life-giving nutrients to every cell in the body and flush the system of waste matter. Pretty incredible stuff. Yet nine times out of ten, humans get hold of this amazing food product, stick it in a pan, heat it to death, cover it with loads of drug-like sugar, sprinkle on some drug-infested cocoa, give it some pretentious French name and call themselves 'Master' chefs. We are the only creatures on the planet that turn something highly nutritious into something detrimental to our health and then brag about being 'masterful' because we have managed to do such a thing.

However, there is one thing that humans have done with fruit and veg which can only be described as truly masterful. Using the enzymes and live nutrients found in all fruit and veg, they have managed to produce something which is even more effective for fat removal and the feeding of every cell in the body than the ultimate fat-busting health pill. What I am talking about here is the ultimate in fast food and nutrient technology. It is the single most powerful fat-blasting, colon-cleansing, nutrient-packed weapon known to man (or woman) kind. No false hunger can possibly survive when you are *mentally* equipped with knowledge of the food trap and *physically* armed with...

29

The Fastest Food in the West

The amazing life-giving, energy-releasing, fat-blasting powers of freshly extracted fruit and vegetable juices are without question the single most powerful and fastest way to get live nutrients through your clogged system and into every cell in your body. It's like employing a super-fast nutrient courier bike to weave in and out of all the built-up traffic to deliver the liquid life-force directly to where it's needed. If you want a sure-fire way to ensure your cells get fed the nutrients they need every day in the fastest and most efficient way it's time to use the fastest nutrient carrier service in the world. When live nutrients positively have to be delivered to your cells on time –

Send it N.P.S. and consider it done

Juicing is the ultimate 'Nutrient Power Service' for your body and there is simply no chemically-manufactured pill, 'nutritious' shake, processed food, canned fruit, bottled or carton juice that comes anywhere near the nutrient power service supplied by freshly extracted fruit and vegetable juices.

Juicing is a truly masterful way of supplying your body with the energy and nutrients it's been crying out for – in the *fastest* possible time and without the energy-zapping digestive process. I will repeat again that it takes more energy to digest food than any other single activity (apart from sex if you recall) and it takes *energy* to get slim and healthy. If you already have a clogged, fat and tired system your body can do with all the help it can get on the digestion front. Shipping your nutrients N.P.S. is a *guaranteed* way of feeding your cells without the body having to go through the very tiring and time consuming process of trying to break it down into usable fuel and then trying to dispose of the leftover waste. The juicing machine does the work that your body normally has to do. It extracts the nutrients from the fruit and veg and disposes of the waste in what's called a 'pulp jug'.

Fruit and some veg are easy for the body to digest, use and dispose of anyway but what makes juicing them so wonderful for an already tired and abused system, is that it takes even *less* work and time for the body to get what it needs from juice. When we *eat* vegetables and fruits the body uses energy trying to squeeze the liquid it needs from the fibre. Guess what? When you put fruit and vegetables through a juicing machine – you've effectively done the body's work for it. By drinking the freshly extracted juice you have skipped the digestive process and efficiently furnished your cells with tons of live nutrients. What many people don't realize is that although vegetables like carrots, broccoli, beetroot, swede, etc. contain tremendous life-giving nutrients that are of huge benefit to our cells and immune system, they are not always easy to get at. In fact the body can have a tough time trying to break down hard veg like carrots and broccoli, especially when it is already tired and weak. This is why we tend to steam or cook them to make them easier to digest. The problem with this, as you will recall, is that when you apply any kind of heat you kill a large percentage of the live nutrients and at the same time *increase* the waste that needs to be disposed of. Juicing is a completely different ball game. The juicing machine breaks down the hard vegetables for you, it then sucks out the live nutrition and puts it in a liquid form that is extremely easy for the body to use.

Fruit is a lot easier for the body to break down than hard vegetables. Whole fruits only take 30 minutes to leave the stomach which, compared to any concentrated food, is extremely fast. Juice, however, is even faster. Juice is on the 15-minute express service, making it by far the fastest food in the west (east, south and north). Nutrients begin to flow through your bloodstream within minutes. Not only that, but only a tiny percentage of these powerful nutrients needs to be used by the body for digestion and disposal. This leaves a *surplus* of raw energy in the body (something it probably won't have had for years). What can the body use this surplus raw energy for? Well it all depends on the individual and what state of health they are in. But, in the majority of people I see, the body uses this extra energy and new superb nutrient workforce to BREAK DOWN AND GET RID OF THE MOUNDS OF EXCESS FAT AND GUNK FROM INSIDE THEIR BODY. It also uses it to help repair your heart, liver, kidneys or whatever other organ or tissue has been badly beaten up for years. All fruit and veg come with their own digestive enzymes. As the body needs very little of these to digest freshly extracted vegetable juice, any leftovers help to digest the concentrated foods we do eat – excellent. And because you have freed your body of so much work, the extra energy saved gets passed on to you. This means tons more raw energy in your daily account to spend however you see fit.

LIQUID GOLD

In terms of 'life' for the body and mind, let me make it quite clear – a daily intake of juice is like the largest ever lottery win. The biggest difference with this lottery is that all you have to do is simply buy your juicing ticket every day and you are GUARANTEED TO WIN. And in terms of true wealth, all the money in the world becomes totally meaningless if your body's enzyme (life) bank account is overdrawn. This type of overdraft can manifest itself in many, many ways: headaches, lethargy, rapid ageing, a clogged system, stored fat, a lack of energy, heart disease, cancer, diabetes, arthritis and asthma – to name but a few. This affects the way you look, think, breath, work and play. In other words, it affects every single thing you do. In terms of sheer quality of life we need to replenish our enzyme account every day. As Dr A. Rosenberger puts it:

**'You lose enzymes through stress, alcohol and processed foods.
You can't get them back from Diet Coke, hot dogs or coffee. You can *only*
replace them with raw, wholefoods – including juices.'**

I am not exaggerating when I say that juicing is quite simply liquid
gold for your body and mind. Every time you drink a glass of freshly
extracted fruit or vegetable juice you can literally feel the goodness
pouring through your system within minutes. It's like injecting a brand
new workforce into your body whose mission is to blast out the fat and
gunk, promote supreme health and give you a new lease of life. And
the taste of the juice you make yourself is in a different league from
the nutritionally-dead versions you see on supermarket shelves
masquerading as the real, 'pure' thing. Even vegetable juice, when
made in the right way, tastes incredible. Of all people I can't believe
I'm saying that. Me, Mr – I would rather stick hot pokers in my eyes all
night than eat broccoli – Vale, is now enthusing about how wonderful
vegetable juice tastes.

The fact is that most people have never tasted freshly extracted
vegetable juice and it's the idea more than anything that's off-putting.
Plus, of course, most people don't know the right way to make
vegetable juices – some of the versions I have tried tasted just a few
rats short of sewer water. But I can assure you that when you taste
just how smooth and creamy they *can* be (the Juice Master way) you
will be converted for life. But as far as I'm concerned even if they
tasted disgusting, given the amazing change in my weight, health and
thinking, I would just hold my nose and pour the stuff down.
Fortunately they do taste incredible and even the ones I found a bit
strange at first, I now love.

THE FUTURE'S BRIGHT, THE FUTURE'S ORANGE (AND GREEN)

We all know that vegetables contain incredible amounts of
antioxidants (blah, blah, blah), which help us build a strong immune
system. The dark green ones like broccoli, spinach and kale contain
something called chlorophyll (nice name). This stuff is simply
sunshine for your cells. Chlorophyll traps the energy of sunlight and

when the plant is broken down the energy is released – this is the best form of carbohydrate known to mankind. The antioxidants and chloro-whatsit found in vegetables all help to *drastically* decrease our chances of getting cancer, heart disease and God knows how many other diseases. This is all excellent. However, for most of us, the idea of sitting down to a plate full of raw broccoli, kale, spinach, celery and carrots doesn't exactly make us want to do somersaults in the snow. In fact, the average person's daily intake of raw live nutrition in the form of fruit and veg is somewhere between 0 and 5 per cent – that pretty much equals suicide! So here's where juicing once again comes into its own.

IF YOU CAN'T EAT THE STUFF – DRINK IT

There is just no way on this planet with my busy schedule that I could get an adequate amount of easy-to-digest nutrients circulating in my system if I didn't juice vegetables every day. I am not a great raw broccoli, kale, celery or beetroot lover and for me juicing them is a very neat way of getting the amazing goodness into my body without having to eat them raw. We are, remember, primarily *fruit-eating* primates and root vegetables are hard for our bodies to break down and use. But if we drink them instead we are doing our bodies a massive favour and helping to 'free up' even more raw energy. At the same time we have, for once, used our incredible know-how to gain access to the live nutrients in hard vegetables without putting a burden on our digestive system.

'I know that if I do not drink a sufficient quantity of fresh raw vegetable juices every day then, as likely as not, my full quota of nourishment enzymes is missing from my body.'

Dr Norman Walker

Dr Walker died peacefully in his sleep, disease *free*, at the age of 113. Another US doctor whose diet also consisted of large quantities of fruit and vegetable juice died at the age of 96 but, to be fair, he didn't die of natural causes like Dr Walker. He was killed by a freak wave whilst surfing. Yes surfing at 96 years of age – that's my kind of guy.

GREEN, GREEN, GREEN

Jay Kordich, *the* juice man in the US, is well known for his statement: 'All life on earth emanates from the green of the plant.' The late Dr Bircher-Benner, who founded the famous Bircher-Benner clinic said, 'There is nothing more therapeutic on earth than green juice'. If there was ever a time to go green now is it. Fruit juices are fab, make no mistake, but it's the green ones that will really supply pure sunshine to every living cell in your body in the fastest way possible, and make a truly unbelievable impact on your health, looks and energy levels – which really can make others green with envy.

What do Goldie Hawn, Gwyneth Paltrow, John F Kennedy, Sean Connery, Madonna, Donna Karan, Nastassja Kinski and Ross Mansergh have in common? Yep you guessed it – JUICE, usually of the veggie kind. Ross Mansergh has perhaps the most remarkable story when it comes to juice. Ross who? Yes not many people have heard of this remarkable man. He is (as the headline read)…

The miracle man who beat cancer with carrots

Well carrot juice to be more specific, with a few apples, leeks and red cabbages thrown in for good measure. He went through 75lbs of carrots a week, 60 apples, six red cabbages and 25lbs of leeks. In his own words, 'The best way to beat cancer is not to poison the body further, but by feeding it the right nutrients'.

He now feels fitter and healthier than he has in years. He no longer needs 75lbs of carrots a week but still gets through at least 15–20lb. Why? Because the best way to *prevent* cancer and heart disease (the two biggest killers by far) is to feed the body the right nutrients on a *regular* basis. If you don't, the live cells which rely on nutrients and oxygen will be slowly starving to death. The huge amount of fruit and veg Ross juiced every week also illustrates how meaningless the 'calorie counting' business is. When he was on his anti-cancer juice regime he was drinking 5,000 calories a day for two years. Yet he never ended up the size of the Napa Valley; in fact he lost some weight and it made him fitter.

You may not be surprised to hear that the 'expert' doctors questioned about this case were not convinced. Dr Ian Smith, consultant at the Royal Marsden Hospital in London, called the treatment 'scientifically unproven'. UNPROVEN? The man's alive and spankingly well. What more proof do you need? Science is 'that which works' and this clearly worked. There is at least one doctor I know of who cannot say enough about the power of juice – Dr Charles Innes. He is 100 per cent convinced that carrot juice saved his life by fighting a brain tumour he had and is even more certain that it stopped him going blind. But the majority of doctors are dismissive of the idea that juicing can have this kind of impact. I have had many 'experts' tell me that some of my theories are 'scientifically unproven', but I am living proof that what I do works and there are many thousands more out there who can testify to the remarkable effects of freeing yourself of the need to eat crap, and the physical raw energy gained by getting juiced every day.

Juicing isn't some kind of new fad either, it's been around for a while. Using raw vegetable juice for healing goes back to the 19th century. At that time of course they didn't have electronic juicing machines. No, back then if you wanted a juice you had to squeeze crushed or chopped vegetables through muslin – a process which took a flipping eternity. Do you think that anyone would have gone through that amount of grief and hassle to make juice if it did no more for a person than the whole vegetable? Never in a million years. Vegetable juice is very nutritious and has an extremely powerful effect on disease of any kind. Max Gerson MD found that when he put his fifty cancer patients on a juice therapy regime all recovered through his natural 'gentle' treatment of cancer (for further details see his book *A Cancer Therapy: Results of Fifty Cases*).

The spark of mental and physical energy you will feel once you are mentally free and physically juiced has a wonderful knock-on effect that helps to change literally every aspect of your life. It not only helps you free yourself of the disease of being fat, tired and lethargic, but also helps you to free yourself of another disease which is sweeping our nation. Nearly every person who walks into my seminars suffers from it in one form or another and it is spreading fast. It is a disease which affects every muscle, cell and organ in your body. It affects your circulation, your breathing, your energy levels, the way you look and the way you feel. It is an insidious disease which affects the shape, tone and muscle structure of your body. It is, of course...

30

Furniture Disease

 'What disease?' Furniture disease – the disease you get from sitting or laying around on various bits of furniture for too long. And boy we do a hell of a lot of it.

As mad as this may sound, a lot of our time is spent sitting on various bits of furniture, usually staring at more bits of furniture. Your average Brit now watches some four to six hours of television a day. That's about 28 hours a week. At that rate if they live till they're 80 they would have spent at least 10 YEARS of their one and only life sitting on furniture watching furniture. I'm not saying don't watch TV (I couldn't live without *Friends*), just that we often don't realize just how little we move our bodies and just how much modern technology has contributed to our lack of oxygen. The average child in the US now spends 21 hours a week watching TV – that's one and half months of TV a year (and what happens there soon happens in the UK). And whilst they're watching the box they'll be subjected to thousands of TV commercials – of which the majority will be for food. Double whammy.

Personally I love the new 'techno toys', it means we can now do things a hell of lot faster than ever before – but it has also brought with it an unbelievable increase in lethargy. We have become so 'advanced' that from the time we wake up to the time we go to sleep we can run our lives from the comfort of our armchairs. Even the shopping can now be done by sitting on furniture tapping your fingers on more furniture. We can order everything from the internet if we wish and have it delivered to our door. Our bills can be paid without us having to leave our chair with the help of telephone banking and the internet. All of this is just fab, but it also means that our bodies are slowly being starved of a good supply of oxygen. Junk and drug food clog the system, as you now realize, but at least we used to have to actually get up and walk to get the stuff. Now we don't even need to get out of our car to reach for a Big Mac or BK Flammer – we can just 'drive through'. In fact for many brands of drug food we haven't even got to leave the house. When I was fat and lethargic and well and truly mentally stuck in the food trap, pizza seemed like a godsend. All I had to do was pick up the phone, oh and go to the door to pay – which at the time seemed like a lot of effort!

When it came to furniture disease, I was no amateur. I mean I had it down to a tee. Play football, are you mad? I can of course play it on Sega! Go skiing? Don't be silly, not when you can pretend on screen. I used to sit up all night some weekends puffing on fags, drinking beer, eating drug foods and playing computer games till daylight with my friends; oh what fun – not! I knew exactly what all the characters in the soap operas were doing, but what was I doing? Not a lot. In fact, many hours of my day was spent watching fictitious characters leading fictitious lives on television whilst chucking dose after dose of drug food down my throat.

So am I saying never use telephone banking, the internet, delivery services, computer games or watch television? NO, NO, NO, of course not. I use all of these and where would I be without my weekly fix of *Frasier*? I am just saying that if you want a level of health that so many people simply *wish* they could have, you need to move your body. The human body is an incredible vehicle, but even the finest fuel in the world will only do so much. As we are all too aware, this fine vehicle of ours was designed to be driven. That is exactly what this book is all about – how to mentally and physically get a light, slim and ENERGY-DRIVEN body. And there is no question that quitting drug foods, cutting back on the junk foods and eating and drinking fruit, veg and their juices, will go a long, long way to getting you that body. However, there is just one more vital ingredient to The Juice Master's recipe for health success. This is a substance which the body needs much more than even the finest foods or juices. It is worth reminding ourselves of the fact that…

You can go weeks without food, days without water, but only minutes without oxygen

An abundance of oxygen is vital for the life of our cells, and I am not talking here about just the shallow incorrect breathing we do every day or the amount we get from just walking up a flight of stairs. That amount of oxygen keeps us going – just. Athletes are something like nine times less likely to get cancer than 'normal' people. What do they do a lot more of than most people? That's right – MOVE. And when they move they *breathe* in a certain manner which feeds tons more life-giving, fat-blasting, blood-circulating, energy-producing oxygen to the cells. By doing this on a regular basis they also automatically keep their lymphatic system free from the build up of billions of cells that are dying every second in the body.

BECOME A LYMPHOMANIAC

What exactly is your lymphatic system? It's a network of vessels that carry lymph – or tissue-cleansing fluid – into the circulatory system. Basically, lymph transports nutrients to the cells and carries away waste products such as dead cells. The system relies on a good supply and flow of oxygen to pump lymph around the body. We have four times more lymph fluid in our body than blood. The blood has its own pump (our heart), but to keep the lymph fluid cleansed it is essential we keep it flowing with the power of deep breath. A good supply of oxygen created by breathing in a certain way cleans the lymph system out.

It's amazing what happens when you breathe properly:
Breathing Restores Energy And Total Health

This doesn't happen for most of us because we are the only creatures in the world that suffer from furniture disease. If we just moved a bit (well a lot), the lymphatic system could just get on with its job and we would feel good. The fact is the human body was designed to MOVE and unless we drive our magnificent vehicle we are slowly starving our body and mind every day of the single most vital ingredient of them all – OXYGEN.

Often when we feel tired and hungry it is as a direct result of not moving enough. The system becomes clogged and the cells begin to be starved of what they need most – a good blast of oxygen. Have you ever felt tired and hungry at the end of the working day, but made the decision to go for a blast down the gym instead of just sitting down and eating? (Okay it might have been some time ago now.) Have you noticed that when you've finished your workout you are less hungry and certainly nowhere near as tired as you were before you started? This is because you have given your body what it thrives on and what it was being deprived of more than anything else – oxygen. I must point out that I am not talking here about walking for 10 minutes on a treadmill whilst thinking about the extra 'points' you are earning. That obviously only adds to a false mental desire and false physical hunger. I am talking about when you move your body until you sweat. 'Hang on Mr Juice Master, I can hear where this oxygen talk is going. Arghhhhhhh –

EXERCISE
(Now there's a sod of a word if ever I heard one)

Um exercise, you know I just hate the word, and it's another favourite of 'The State The Bleeding Obvious Brigade' who regularly informed me, 'You know you really should do more exercise, it would help you lose weight'. Like I hadn't figured this one out for myself. But here was the problem. I was tired, I looked awful and I felt lousy most of the time. Just the idea of running for a hour on a treadmill made me reach for a cream bun! The thought of joining a gym with all those slim people was very daunting – I mean, come on, I was fat. And besides all that, I HATED IT. I'd tried 'exercising' many times and it just wasn't for me – or so I thought.

Just as I could never imagine drinking vegetable juice, eating salad and not eating chocolate, so I would never have thought in a million years that I would feel so juiced that I would *want* to move my body every day. But then that was before I discovered the single most effective and most enjoyable exercise programme in the world. Now you can't stop me doing it – I love it. And as unbelievable as this may sound to you at the moment, you will too.

I actually discovered this exercise programme many years ago but only started to do again after I got juiced. It is one that you may even have done in the past yourself but at the time you simply didn't realize that what you were doing was…

31

The Best
Exercise Programme
in the World

So what exactly is it? Quite simply – THE ONE YOU ENJOY DOING.

It's no good some expert telling me that the best form of exercise for me is to go on the rowing machine for half an hour, because I hate it. So I won't do it. You can have the finest exercise machine in the world but if it bores the pants off you you're not going to use it. It is therefore *not* a good exercise programme for you.

'Can young Johnny come out to burn some calories please?'

You won't hear that – ever. Children 'exercise' all the time (although with the new techno toys it's getting less and less) but they don't call it exercise, they say can we go and play. They don't give two hoots whether they are playing aerobically or anaerobically, they just enjoy playing. The mental energy you gain from feeling free from the food trap and the physical energy you gain from sending your live fuel N.P.S. every day will give you that spark again to go and play.

I went to a very big seminar some years ago in the States. On sale was a machine that was being hailed as, you guessed it, the best exercise programme in the world. This machine gave 'the ultimate workout' in just four minutes The cost? TEN THOUSAND DOLLARS.

I had a go – and had about as much fun as I would plucking my nasal hairs with a fish fork! For me the machine was about as effective as a cat-flap in a hippo's house. It's bad enough when you watch the dust settling on the running, rowing or home exercise bike which cost a few hundred quid, but can you imagine owning a $10,000 machine that you only ever use for a few days every new year?

The best exercise programme in the world is one that's enjoyable and fun – for *you*. If someone got on that $10,000 machine and loved it, had fun on it, had the money, then magic – they have found something that works for them. Luckily for me I found something which costs an average of £10. It's called a football. All I need is a ball, a park and I'm as happy as pie. And if there's a goal with a net still up in it then I'm quite simply in heaven. I also love tennis, squash, rounders, aerobics, cycling, table tennis, swimming, water polo, basketball, running, water pistol fighting and trampolining.

The way you move your body determines how you feel, how you feel often determines what you put into your body, what you put into your body determines how you feel

The reason why I didn't 'exercise' in the past wasn't because I was lazy. It was because I wasn't physically or mentally juiced. I didn't like 'exercise' so I wasn't *mentally* inspired, but I did like having fun. My only problem was that I was simply out of practice on the physical, fun side of things.

You can get rid of all the drug foods and drinks and feed your body with tons of super-fast nutrition, but unless you are mentally inspired to move your body, you will still suffer from a lack of oxygen to the cells – otherwise known as furniture disease.

There is no such thing as laziness, just an uninspired mind

You tell any lazy, so-called couch potato that they've just won £12m on the lottery – see how they move then. So what am I saying? That we need a lottery win every day to make us move our bodies? NO (although it would be nice). I am saying that we just need to find something that will *mentally* inspire us to move our body. Look at children – the minute they see snowfall they're running, leaping, throwing snowballs, making sledges from baking trays and having lots of FUN. When it snows it stimulates a 'lottery-win' chemical reaction in the mind of the child (or adult). They smile more, laugh more, feed oxygen to their brain and cells, and get all the exercise they need without ever calling it exercise. They build up an incredible appetite, so enjoy their food more and, afterwards, they sleep like a baby. Not only that, they also interact with others, make more friends and expand their lives. Somehow running on a treadmill in your house doesn't quite hit all the same notes, but finding the best exercise programme in the world for *you*, gives you all those things and more every single day.

We often put our reluctance to play down to our age, or a lack of time (always a good one), but that doctor I mentioned earlier was still surfing when he was 96 years old. He died doing 'The Best Exercise Programme In The World' – for him. There is just no question that surfing gave that man much, much more than just physical exercise. And there is no question that when you start to move your body in a way that stimulates your mind and body, it will give you so much more than just a slim body. Physical movement improves your daily quality of life in so many different ways. Not only does it feed your body and mind with the life-giving, fat-blasting, energy-*increasing* oxygen it so desperately craves, it makes you feel lighter, happier and more relaxed. You sleep better, think clearer, have more energy and get such incredible pleasure from ending a genuine hunger that even your meal times are a complete joy. That's not all, when you play – instead of 'exercise' – your body produces anti-cancer chemicals. I kid you not, there is a man in the US who managed, with the help of laughter, to beat his cancer. This illustrates why walking on a treadmill, stressed out of your head is not really the best way of getting yourself moving – although it's better than a clip around the ear with a wet kipper. FUN, FUN, FUN – that's the key. If you *enjoy* the feeling you get from a good blast on the treadmill – then do it.

Children love to play and if truth be known so do we. In reality we are all kids who happen to play at being an adult most of the time.

Kids come back from school and they just *want* to play. I'm now back in the position where I am so mentally and physically juiced that when I've finished work I too want to go and play. I am now disappointed if for some reason I *can't* go to the park or the gym – and that's somewhat of a turn around I can tell you.

I have more mental and physical energy now than I can ever remember having in my adult life and more importantly I have more FUN in my life now. I often don't even wait until after work to go and play – as soon as I wake up I put my favourite music on and jump up and down on my mini trampoline or put on my KanGoo boots and bounce around the park like Zebedee. Am I mad? Probably, but I love it, and it's much better than waking up uninspired, tired, lethargic, groggy and reaching for a coffee to give me a false kick-start.

Do you remember bouncing on the bed when you were a kid? Wasn't it fun? Do you remember dancing in your room to your favourite tune just for the fun of it? Do you remember playing football, hockey, squash, netball, rounders, badminton, or tennis? Do you remember how much fun roller skates were? What about games in the pool as a kid or games in the street which required just physical movement and pure un*adult*erated imagination? Four things all of them had in common – they all required physical exercise, they were all fun, they all made you totally oblivious to any problems you thought you had and perhaps the most important thing – they all made you feel good. When you move your body to the point where you sweat it just makes you feel so good. And isn't that what we are all working so hard to achieve – just to *feel* good? Maybe it's not a lottery win we need, or a promotion, but simply some team games, some physical movement, a bit of stimulating music and some fun. In fact, if you think about it, some of the best nights in or out seem to involve some kind of physical movement until we sweat (I was actually talking about dancing – well maybe).

Does this mean that a nice long walk in the country is no good for you, that you have to be bouncing around every two minutes in order to get some benefit? No. Any kind of physical movement (especially if it's outdoors) is fantastic. There aren't many things as nice or as therapeutic as a long walk in the woods or along a beach. But in order to really supply your already starved body with some dynamic fuel at the same time as having fun, you really do need to find the best exercise programme in the world – and do it till you sweat.

We are not talking here about just one thing either, the beauty of the best exercise programme in the world is that it could be many different things to you depending on the day, the weather, the people you are with etc. All these factors will play a part in determining exactly which physical movement I am going to do on any particular day. If it's a sunny morning, I will head for the park with my football or go outside and jump on my mini trampoline. If it's raining, I'll do a high-powered aerobics class at the gym. Yes me, Mr – I'd rather stamp idiot on my forehead than do aerobics – Vale, doing aerobics at 7am and loving it.

IF MUSIC BE THE FOOD OF OXYGEN – PLAY ON

Have you ever been out for dinner with a group of friends and felt too tired to go dancing afterwards? In the end you go because everyone else is bugging you to. But then what happens? One of your favourite tunes comes on and BOOM – you're shaking your tail feather! The more you move your body the more alive you become – why? Because you are feeding oxygen to your cells, getting an adrenaline surge and having fun. People just come alive when they are doing something which is fun for them. You've done God knows how much 'physical exercise' but because it was fun, you never called it exercise and it never felt like exercise. I also believe that music has something to do with it. The best music in the world is an unbelievable stimulus for getting you moving. What is the best music in the world? The one *you* love, the one that gets *you* going, the one that inspires *you*. I have made a mini-disc of all the tunes that inspire me, the ones *I* love, and whatever physical movement I am doing alone, I stick on my headphones and BOOM – it's ten times more fun. Jumping up and down on my mini trampoline is fun, but add some funky music and it just increases the pleasure ten fold.

JUST DO IT

Whatever you choose on any given day to be the best exercise programme in the world for you, make sure you go beyond just *knowing* what it is – **do it**. After all by simply 'joining' a gym you get nothing. You will find that even if you hate the idea of a gym and can never envisage liking anything it has to offer, just like 'changing your brand' of food, it will soon be a part of your life you couldn't imagine being without... I now actually like running on a treadmill to music – it gives me time to think and de-stress after a hard day, and I feel so blooming great afterwards. So even if at first you don't particularly like 'exercising' at the gym, you will soon be hooked. Thirty per cent of people who join a gym stop going in the first month and that figure goes up to a whopping 80 per cent after just three months. Some people continue paying every month for years, yet never go. My gym has over 2000 members, yet you see the same 20 people every night. There are two main reasons why people who find what they enjoy, then fail to actually do it. One is that their body can sometimes be so tired from a lifetime of abuse that they physically cannot participate. In this case a few weeks free from the food trap and the help of some super-charged juice will make them feel lighter and give them a better opportunity to at least slowly join in the fun. The second reason why people fail to do the physical acts that they would love to do is by far the most common. It is caused by an awful phobia that seems to be on the increase. Virtually everyone I meet in my seminars has suffered from it at various times and there
is no question it prevented them participating. It is so insidious that it can stop people swimming, playing rounders, beach volleyball, doing aerobics, dancing and ever having sex (oh we must get rid of this one).

You will have no problem whatsoever enjoying the best exercise programme in the world to the fullest once you are not just free from the food trap and physically juiced, but also totally free from...

32

People Phobia

People what? Phobia! A truly life- and soul-destroying phobia
that can, and so often does, prevent people from doing what
they would love to do. More importantly it is the very thing
that can prevent you from doing the best exercise programme in the
world. However, once you get this baby licked, your quality of life will
explode and you will feel freer than you've felt in years.

SO WHAT IS PEOPLE PHOBIA?

People phobia is when you are so worried about what other people
may think of you that it stops you from truly living. I used to suffer
from this phobia – big time. It was hardly surprising when you
consider that I was fat, had bigger breasts than your average supermodel and was covered from head to toe in psoriasis. I used to cover
myself with two towels before jumping into a swimming pool; I would
keep my top on a hot summer's day, even if I was sweating cobs (as
they say); if I ever did go to the gym I would come home to shower
and change, despite the fact they had showers, steam-rooms and
saunas at the gym; and I always kept the lights very low or off at 'bed'
time (if you catch my drift). But I realize now that I did all of those
things, not because I was fat or my skin was bad, but because I was

suffering from 'people phobia'. After all, would I have kept my top on if I was by myself and there wasn't a soul in sight? Would I have wrapped two towels around my body if it were my own private pool? Would I have gone home in my sweaty clothes after a session in the gym if it was my gym and I was alone? NO WAY! I would have felt free to be me. And that's what I am talking about here, being truly mentally free.

How on earth can we ever be truly free to do what we want if we are constantly worrying about what other people may or may not think of us? The bottom line is we can't. Unless we nip this in the bud *now* people phobia can stop you from sucking the juice from life and living a truly free and playful life. Life is just too short to ever have to suffer from what is a pretty egotistical way to think anyway – yes egotistical! When I was fat and lethargic I certainly never considered myself in anyway egotistical, I mean what the hell did I have to be egotistical about? But if we don't do things we would love to do for fear of what others may think of us, then we must have not just egos, but super egos. What makes us think we are so special that everyone's going to look and talk about us? And what makes us think that even if they are making a comment about us that it is in some way negative? And quite frankly who gives a flying care if it is? If they are the kind of people who are that critical and judgmental you don't want to be associated with them anyway. The truth is that most people just aren't looking at you and couldn't care less what you are doing or how you look. How often have you looked at someone that was a bit different? Do you continue staring and talking about them 24 hours a day? NO! You look, think about it for a millisecond and just get on with your life. So why do we think that just because we happen to a bit fatter, thinner, older or out of step, that everyone is going to be talking about us? Get it clear – THEY'RE NOT! Yes they may look, but then don't we all tend to look at someone new? In fact don't we just tend to look – period. It's what we do; it's why hidden cameras and fly-on-the-wall documentaries are so popular – people like watching people. The problem only lies in the way *we* are thinking about ourselves. If you believe you're too fat, too old, too whatever, you are always going to believe that everyone else is also thinking about you in the same way, but it's time to realize THEY DON'T CARE. When I was overweight and had an unsightly skin disease I was so paranoid I believed 'they' were judging me, yet I now know that most people in a gym actually admire anyone who comes and has a go, especially if they are fat. They tend to look in admiration, and anyone who looked at my skin problem was looking out of concern – not revulsion. I am free from the stupid egotistical belief that the world is looking at me and talking about me. We need to realize the problem is not what other people are thinking, but what *we* believe they are thinking and the fact we allow this to alter our behaviour. It is *our* thinking that is the problem – not theirs. If we change the way we think, the problem simply cannot exist.

'Poor is the man whose pleasure depends on the permission of another'
(Madonna – surprisingly)

People phobia can prevent you from doing just about anything: dancing the way that expresses who you are, joining a gym, doing aerobics, sunbathing, wearing certain clothes, going swimming – and yes, if you are paranoid about your weight, your age, your skin etc. it can even stop you having sex.

I don't want anything to get in the way of your success and part of that success comes from giving yourself permission to go out and play again – it's the very essence of the best exercise programme in the world. Many people would love to join a gym but don't do it because they think everyone will look at them. They're worried about not being able to keep up or do the right steps and movements in an aerobics class. They're concerned what people will think of them if they don't have the right clothes. They're worried about the shape of their body or whether they're going to fit in. How do I know? Because that's exactly how I felt for years – right up until the point where I realized that it just didn't matter. I remember stepping into my local gym some eight years ago now to do my first ever aerobics class with Mad Theo from L.A. Gym in Peckham. Not only had I never done aerobics, but I was fat, I was new and I was a man. In fact, apart from the instructor, I was the only man in there. But I just didn't care any more, I'd heard from a friend that this class was fun (key word) and I actually felt mentally free to just do it. What I didn't realize was that I had walked in to perhaps the highest impact class ever devised. I did all the wrong moves, stood out a mile and had to stop quite a few times as I wasn't the fittest cookie in the biscuit barrel. But the music was good, I was having fun and it felt good. Then I had the added advantage of everyone in the class liking me – why? Because I made everyone look fantastic! I was the most out-of-step, out-of-shape person in there and they loved having me there.

A woman in her seventies sent me a beautiful letter a couple of months after attending one of my seminars. She explained how her life had completely changed since she'd not only freed herself from the food trap, but of her people phobia. She had started line dancing in her mid-seventies, had met loads of wonderful people and made many new friends – and she feels younger, fitter and freer than she has felt in years. In her words, 'I feel like a child again and I love it'.

It is such a cliché to say it but it is so true – we get one life and we cannot afford not to live it to the full because of pointless worrying about what people (most of whom we have never met) may think of what we are doing. Who cares what they think? NOT ME, that's for sure. Young children don't care either. In fact by watching them we can learn so much. Children tend to live by two very simple rules and if you follow them BOOM – no more phobia. Children –

Move like they can't be seen *and* sing like they can't be heard

No wonder they only need a pop song, or some snow to be happy.

Whenever you hit a situation where you would have previously worried about people looking at you or judging you, simply walk, talk, breathe and move like you are the only person there – and quietly smile to yourself. (People in their cars at traffic lights who pick their noses seem to have this off to a tee). What I am talking about is a frame of mind where you simply do things freely, where you are free to be you and free to play: a frame of mind that allows you to walk around the pool without the towels wrapped around you, one that allows you to dance and act a bit silly when you want and one which allows you to join that class and not give two hoots if you're a little bit out of step. If you do happen to do an aerobics class, stand at the front and just feel how liberating it is. Wear the brightest colours if you want to – if you are going to stand out at least do it in style. In my seminars I play loud music and give people a chance to dance like they can't be seen, to move as if they are the only ones in the room. Even some of the biggest, shyest and most insecure people are rocking and rolling in no time. They can't get the moves wrong, because there are no rules – it's total freestyle. They are moving their bodies in front of a room of people like they haven't done in years – and they love it.

WHO WANTS TO BE A SLIMIONAIRE?

One young man who attended a recent seminar springs to mind when it comes to this subject – his name is Terry. He was severely people phobic and as such lacked a hell of a lot of confidence. He was also fairly big and well and truly stuck in the food trap. It was, as I was informed later, an incredible achievement just to get him to attend – but I am so pleased he did. Terry went from strength to strength as the day went on. Not only was he soon dancing, but his name was picked to play the Juice Master's *Who Wants To Be A Slimionaire?* This incredible young man not only got up and took centre stage in front of a room full of strangers, but he played full-out! The audience also played their part and for various reasons it was one of those special moments you never forget.

He continued to play full-out throughout the day and at the end of the seminar his sister explained that the change in a day was nothing short of remarkable. Terry was virtually in tears at the end and finished by saying, 'From now on I'm going to move like I can't be seen and sing like I can't be heard. I was a little out of step a few times there, but you know what... it really doesn't matter does it? Thank you, I feel free'. There is simply no question that that man's life is going to totally change. He is going to have more joy, more fun and feel freer than he has ever felt in his adult life. This in turn will have a knock-on effect on his relationships, his work, his ambitions, his dreams – in fact to every aspect of his entire one and only life.

So if you want to join a gym – go do it. If you want to jump on a pair of roller-blades regardless of your age or weight – go do it. If you want to pick up a hair brush and sing to Elvis and wiggle your hips in the mirror – go do it. If you want to jump on a mini-trampoline to some funky music – go do it. If you haven't been to a club for years and you're in the mood to have a boogie – just go do it. If you want to go hiking in the Lake District – go do it. In fact whatever you want to do – GO DO IT. And do it TODAY. If you feel free from the start you *are* free from the start. And that is what this whole book is about – your freedom.

It's about freedom to move in a way you haven't done in years; freedom to eat and drink life-giving, fat-blasting foods and drinks everyday; freedom to flood your system with liquid gold; freedom from the need to consume drug foods; freedom to wear what you want when you want. Freedom to be with other people eating drug foods and not envy what they are doing but, for the first time ever, genuinely pity them for the poor drug food addicts they are; total freedom to be yourself every day no matter who is there or what you may look like; freedom to enjoy the process of becoming slim and energy-driven; freedom to do the best exercise programme in the world whenever you want; freedom from the diet industry for the rest of your life; freedom from 'people phobia' and freedom from the life-destroying FOOD TRAP forever. I am talking about being and feeling totally free. That is exactly how I feel – FREE.

This kind of freedom is yours for the taking and the only thing that can possibly prevent you from getting there is fear. But remember, this fear is just yet another symptom of being a drug food addict. Think of the mouse in the cage. The drug had slowly shattered its central nervous system so much that in the end it was fearful of *not* being able to hit the button. Any outsider could clearly see the mouse should have been fearful about continuing to hit it, not stopping. And this is exactly what drug foods and drinks do to people. The key to freedom is not to feel deprived because you are no longer hitting the button, but be totally relieved and euphoric that you have finally stepped out of the cage, set yourself free and are in a position where you no longer have to hit the button ever again.

The reason people feel so gloomy when they're on a diet is because they believe they are 'giving up' something worth having. They go through what amounts to a mental grieving process, as if they have lost some kind of friend. But what kind of friend is it that physically and mentally abuses you every day? What kind of friend shatters your nervous system? What kind of friend undermines your confidence and keeps you their slave? What kind of friend beats you up and then pretends to help you out? What kind of friend demands you feed them at the cost of starving yourself? FRIEND? Who needs enemies? Drug foods and drinks are not your friends, they are your enemy. These so-called pick-me-up friends have been undermining your confidence; taking away your self-respect; keeping you a slave; keeping you an addict; keeping you fat, tired and lethargic; stealing your money; and, behind your back, they have been planning your death. So I wouldn't have any qualms or feel nervous about kicking them out of your life. Drug foods are designed to shatter the central nervous system and create a degree of *false* insecurities and fear – so if you are in any way nervous about the change I would simply feel the *false* fear and starve it to death.

There is nothing to fear from making the change but everything to fear from *not* making it

It is only fear that keeps people hooked on drug foods and drinks. It is only fear that keeps them looking for ways to try and control these nightmare substances instead of just letting go of them completely. It is only fear that prevents them from gaining the quality of life they ultimately crave. Don't allow this false fear to keep you hooked for the rest of your life. That is exactly what these fears are – FALSE. Just like the false pleasure, the false comfort and the false hungers these nightmare substances cause, the fear they create is also very false. I once heard a great acronym for fear:

False Evidence which Appears Real

One which is perhaps equally or more apt in this case would be False Eating which Appears Real. And that is certainly the case here. The fear people have of changing their eating habits *appears* real because of the illusionary effects of the drug foods and drinks. The illusions are giving false evidence which appears real to you. Using the mouse in the cage as an example – the fear of just running out of the cage and being free appeared real to the mouse, but it was false. The drug was causing the feelings of insecurities and dissatisfaction, yet the false evidence indicated the opposite to the mouse. This caused it to fear life without the drug and this is why even though the cage was open it was still trapped – by a *false* feeling of insecurity and fear. And it's exactly this false fear which keeps people rooted in the food trap. But when you open your mind and see behind the brainwashing and through the fear, what is there to fear by making the change? What is there to be scared of? NOTHING! In fact it's all good; there is no down-side whatsoever to breaking free. But what is there to fear by *not* making the change? EVERYTHING!

Fear can hold you prisoner...the truth will set you free

There is no question that if you have understood what I have said so far then total freedom is yours for the taking. All you need to do now is make a very simple choice based on your new-found understanding of the food trap, the best exercise programme in the world, the fastest food in the west and people phobia. You can either carry on as you are for the rest of your one and only short life on this planet, sinking further and further into the trap – getting more lethargic, more overweight, more insecure, more enslaved, more people phobic – OR YOU CAN GET THE HELL OUT ASAP. To put it another way, the choice you have is quite simply this, it is time to either…

33

Get Busy Living or Get Busy Dying

It's your call

I want to make this point very clear: the food trap is like quicksand and unless you get out it will suck you further and further down. You cannot simply sit on the fence when it comes to this decision because there is no fence, it's one or the other – either get busy living or you get busy dying.

THERE IS NO IN-BETWEEN

All drug addiction is a form of disease and slavery, including drug food addiction. And like any disease it doesn't just get better one day and it doesn't just disappear if you ignore it – IT WILL CONTINUE TO GET WORSE. Each day you will become just a little more tired, a little more lethargic, a little more diseased, a little more starved, a little more insecure, a little more hooked, a little more stressed, a little more unhealthy and just a little more overweight. Each day adds to the next and that 'little' soon becomes a hell of a lot. People think they just wake up one day with heart disease, cancer, irritable bowel syndrome, gallstones etc. One day they were fine, the next – BOOM! They then look for what could have caused 'it'. Of course it can't have been their crap diet that caused it, after all they have been eating and drinking the same stuff for years, seemingly with no major life-threatening problem – so naturally it must be genetic. And how do we tend to treat that – with TOXIC DRUGS.

ONE CHOCOLATE BAR HAS NEVER KILLED ANYONE BUT THEN NEITHER HAS ONE CIGARETTE

It's the thousands that go along with it that are the problem. Drug food and drink addiction is a chain reaction, each one creating the false mental and physical need for the next. Each one causes an imbalance in the body chemistry, thus creating *additional* empty feelings which only seem to be filled with more of the same. The more empty drug foods and drinks you consume the larger the void, the larger the void the more you consume – it's a trap. That is why trying to cut down doesn't work, in fact it makes it worse. All you do is exercise *more* control over the very things which are in reality are controlling you. Unless you step outside the cage and see for yourself exactly what's happening and break the chain completely it will continue for the rest of your life and you will *never* be free. If you choose not to open your mind to what's really going on, if you choose *not* to starve out the false fear and the little drug food parasites and leap to freedom, you will spend the rest of your life a slave to drug foods and drinks – being mentally and physically beaten by them daily.

YOUR FUTURE IN THEIR HANDS

Is that what you want? A lifetime of always hating the way you look and feel, never being able to wear what you want when you want: a future which consists of never being able to move the way you want; never experiencing what it's like to have a light, slim and energy-driven body. You will spend the rest of your life on a constant daily diet: always thinking about controlling your intake, always using a degree of willpower and discipline not to 'hit the button' too often, *constantly* trying not to sink any further – that's not living. And if you are not living you are dying – it's that simple.

Most people think you only have two choices: either eat these foods, feel guilty, get unhealthy and fat and wish you hadn't; or exercise willpower and control not to eat them and feel miserable, deprived and envy the people who are eating them. Either way you have a problem. With the foods or without them, you'll be miserable. Imagine having to spend the rest of your life doing this – what a living nightmare. But there is another option and it makes the whole process of getting a slim and energy-driven body so easy. Simply see these so-called foods for what they really are, see behind the advertising and glossy packaging, make a decision to dump them from your life and jump for joy that you are finally free *not* to eat them. Wow, what a concept – a *happy* non-drug-food eater. No more doom and gloom, only total elation at solving your food problem for life.

This is where everyone gets it wrong. It seems the whole world believes that if you *don't* have these nightmare substances flooding your body – making you ill and fat, and controlling your life – you're missing out on something. But there is nothing to miss, it is all one huge confidence trick, one massive illusion. There is nothing to give up, there is no struggle, and freedom from the food trap is easy. It is, after all, very difficult to get depressed or feel deprived when *nothing* has been taken from you. If you've understood what I have said so far it should by now be crystal clear that it's not you who will be missing out or giving up – it's them. It's the poor drug food addict that's missing out on just about everything and they are the ones who are constantly giving up. They're giving up their health, their money, their energy, their life force and their freedom. And all for what? What do they get in return?

NOTHING

I want to make it very clear that all the sacrifices are made when you are eating and drinking these kinds of foods, not when you quit. All the sacrifices are made if you don't have liquid energy flowing through your bloodstream feeding your cells every day. If you are a tired, lethargic, overweight drug food junkie then you make sacrifices in every area of your life – from your physical and mental vibrancy, your health and energy levels to your relationships and the amount you can get out of your life.

IF YOUR LIFE ISN'T EXPANDING – IT'S SHRINKING AND IF YOU'RE NOT LIVING – YOU'RE DYING

I know that no matter what state of health you are in, or how badly addicted you think you are or not, you can *easily* turn everything around. I was a chain-smoking, dope-smoking, heavy-drinking, drug food and drug drink addict who was fat, badly asthmatic, covered from head to toe in psoriasis. I come from a one parent family, I left school at 15 and used to live on a council estate in one of the worst parts of south east London. It doesn't matter where you are at this moment, what you have tried, what you have been through, or what your story is (believe me, we all have a story), it really doesn't have to be hard work or a struggle to make the change. It's simply down to the correct frame of mind. *Not* making the change is hard work. It's *not* doing anything about it that creates tremendous pain. Your present state of health is a direct result of the decisions you've made in the past, but let me make the next point very clear –

The past does not equal the future

If you are driving your car and you want to go forward do you stare in your rear view mirror? Of course not. Remember the past does not equal the future, it's what you do TODAY that counts. So many people carry unwanted failures with them through life, fearing they can't succeed because of what happened yesterday, or last week, or last month, or 10 years ago – RUBBISH. You will succeed and it's easy. Follow the Juice Master's Ultimate Health recipe and a light, slim and energy-driven body is yours for the taking. It doesn't matter how long you've been eating your brand, how much you used to have or how many times you have tried in the past – *anybody* can find it easy and enjoyable to change their brand of food and get moving for life. All you have to do is:

UNDERSTAND THE NATURE OF THE TRAP
AND FOLLOW THE RECIPE

You must get it clear in your mind that all the knowledge in the world is nothing without the final ingredient – ACTION. So many people know what they need to do and sometimes they even know how they can do it, but they fail to actually do it. It's not what you know that counts, it's what you do with what you know. What sets apart the successes from the failures is the ability to take *action*; the ability to go beyond simply *talking* about a good life; the ability to go that one stage further than just *thinking* about the change; the ability to truly decide.

A TRUE DECISION = CERTAINTY
HOPE = UNCERTAINTY

The key to lifelong change is just that – to truly decide. Not to *hope* but to KNOW FOR CERTAIN. If you hope you are going on holiday, it doesn't mean you are going anywhere, but if you know for certain – then you will go for certain. Once you book your place you are as good as there. It's the same with the food trap: it may take a while to shift the physical symptoms left over from being a victim of the food trap for so many years, but the minute you make a concrete decision to follow the recipe – a concrete decision to board the plane to the place I describe as Mauritius – then you are as good as there. Once you make a true decision you cut off any other possibility. That is what decision in its Latin form means: 'to cut off from', 'to terminate'. You remove any other possibility so that whatever happens in your future life, good days or bad, reaching for drug-like food to help with an emotion of any kind is simply not an option. It's the equivalent of turning to heroin in such times, it is something that you simply wouldn't consider because you know it won't actually make the situation better. You have moved on and you are free.

When you make a true decision you give your brain an air of certainty which it thrives on; when you *hope* things will turn out okay you give your brain an air of *uncertainty* which creates doubts, insecurities and fears – and this wears you down. So it's time to stop *talking* supreme health and a slim body – it's time to DECIDE to have it. The minute you decide, really decide *and* have the correct mental and physical recipe to follow – it's yours.

WHATEVER YOUR DECISION IT WILL DETERMINE YOUR FUTURE LIFE

Let's make something very clear, the decision to actually follow the ultimate recipe – to get busy living, to choose health over disease, to choose slim over fat – is without doubt the single most important decision you will ever make in your life. Nothing even comes close to just how important this decision is. You cannot buy your way to the land of the healthy and slim – *you can only do it*. All the money in the world is meaningless if you are tired, lethargic, fat, miserable and constantly battling with drug foods and drinks and your weight. All the money in the world is of no use if you are in the cage. It's no good being a wealthy prisoner is it? The good news is it's *easy* to escape – the door has always been open. You are your own jailer, so make the decision to walk to freedom – it's a decision that will totally change the quality, and very likely the length, of your future life.

Some people say to me, 'Yes but you can get run over by a bus next week' and yes of course you can, but would you take heroin just because you could get run over by a bus next week? OF COURSE YOU WOULDN'T. There is a bus coming along for all of us – it's the daily *quality* of our lives that counts. It is how we feel TODAY. It's making sure that we are in control of our lives *before* the bus comes along that ultimately counts – making certain that we *live* and not simply survive before our bus arrives.

So remember, the past does not equal the future – it's what you do today that counts. The decision to act or not act on the information in this book will determine your future life – sink even further or jump to freedom? I cannot stress enough just how easy it is to change what you eat and how enjoyable it is to get moving again – it's simply down to how you think. And when you look at it, when you really simplify it, it really only comes down to just a couple of things: decide to kick the rubbish foods from your life and don't pine, mope or feel down about your decision – rejoice and jump for joy from the start.

That's it. It really can be that simple. It is only the indecision, the pining, the moping, the counting days and feeling miserable about it that makes it difficult. But what the hell is there to feel down or miserable about? NOTHING. You're *not* going on a diet, you're not going to be avoiding certain situations, your *not* going to be starving yourself, you're *not* putting a stop to dinner parties or going out, in fact you're going to be free to eat, free to move and free to live. Remember –

This is not a diet and this is not a rigid, boring exercise programme. It's total freedom

You can now look forward to a future where you can eat freely, move freely and live freely. So get excited, you are about to get busy living – really living. You are about to go on a journey that will literally *shape* your entire destiny. You are about to use the ultimate mental and physical health recipe that will guarantee you freedom, health and a slim body for life. You will sleep better, think clearer, and feel lighter, sexier and freer than you have in years. Every part of your life will be affected, from your work to your everyday relationships. And you'll find your confidence will explode. It really is hard to put into words how I was and how I am now – the difference really is like night and day. Your food problem is being solved for life and you are off to the land of the slim and healthy – WOW!

At this stage I cannot blame you for being like a dog on a leash, straining to get on with it, dying to just get on the plane. But wait –YES PLEASE WAIT. Before you start your journey you need to be *fully* prepared. You have struggled for years and it's not going to take long to read just a couple more chapters. They could mean the difference between 'Slim and Healthy For A Week' and 'Slim and Healthy For Life'. You need to know exactly what to expect on the journey so that nothing throws you. So to make absolutely certain of your success before I give you *all* of the ingredients that make up The Ultimate Health Recipe in a simplified form, there are a couple of things you need to watch out for. First up it's...

34

The Food Police

Yes – the food police. This is the squad that goes around watching *everything* you eat and drink. These are the people who, knowing you have changed your eating habits, will pick up on anything you eat that's not fresh fruit or vegetables. This is the force that believes you have somehow committed a crime by breaking free from the constant need to eat crap; that you are a do-gooder and it's their job to pick up on any 'normal' foods you do eat and ram it down your throat (figuratively speaking that is). Yes the food police are out there in full force, and on your journey to the land of the slim and healthy, they are all too ready to pounce. In fact it seems even if it's been years since you made the change some just never seem to go away (do they Anna, Tim and Frances) – so be very alert.

You would think that people would be pleased for you if you were out of the cage and no longer hitting the button, especially those closest to you. You would think they would be happy that you have changed what you eat and are on the road to being slim and healthy wouldn't you? Well yes you would think so, but in order to have a pleasant journey there is one thing you must realize when making the change –

Nobody minds you changing what you eat and drink,
nobody minds you going to the gym,
nobody minds you declining a dessert
PROVIDING OF COURSE YOU'RE MISERABLE ABOUT IT!

It's sad, but true. If you are moping around, getting uptight, depressed and moaning that you 'can't' have what you want, then they are fine – in fact they secretly quite like it. But if you are happy about quitting the rubbish – if you are enjoying eating and drinking fresh produce, and loving the journey to the land of the slim and healthy – they hate it.

Why?

Because you are a constant reminder of what they know they should and, in reality, would love to be doing. And every time they see you eating fresh produce and having no desire for drug foods and drinks it makes them feel even worse than they normally feel after consuming rubbish. This leads them to try and justify their reasons for eating and drinking this stuff, and to cries of 'health freak' and even feelings of resentment. This is why they join the food police. They just can't wait for you to commit a 'food crime' so they can slap you with a humiliation fine. They can't wait for you to fail and will often do anything in their power to bully you into changing back, or use their persuasive powers to lure you back.

No drug addict likes to be the only one taking it –
including drug food addicts

If I was offering apples to all my friends and they declined I would have no problem eating one. I wouldn't feel ashamed, I wouldn't call them names or claim they have flaws in their personality because they choose not to have one – would you? Yet with drug foods it's different. If you say no to a dessert, the drug food addicts can't just leave it there. They say things like 'Come on you boring bastard', 'Live a little', 'Stop being so unsociable', 'I remember when you were fun', 'It's only a bit of chocolate, it's hardly going to kill you', 'What's the matter with you?', 'Life's too short', 'You could get run over by a bus tomorrow'. But how on earth does not having a piece of cake make you boring, unsociable, unfunny or mean you're not living any more? If someone doesn't want a grape they don't get this crap do they? They don't have to justify why they *don't* want one. Why? Because grapes are a natural food and we don't feel instinctively stupid eating them. But with drug foods we do. This is why if you do say no to them, the drug food addict will do everything in their power to make sure you 'join them'. If someone else is doing it they feel better – in exactly the same way as a smoker will feel much better smoking in the company of at least one other smoker.

'YOU HEALTH FREAK'

Yes you'll definitely hear this one alright, time and time again. It's without question their favourite: 'You health freak'. You will hear it when you first make the change and to some degree for the rest of your life – and I'm not kidding either. Yes, when all else fails they will try to make themselves feel better about what they are doing by calling you a freak. But I wonder how they'd feel if you responded by calling them a 'Disease Freak'? How on earth does eating well suddenly turn you into a freak? In reality there should be no such thing as a health freak: it shouldn't be seen as 'freaky' to be healthy – it should be totally normal. The fact that it is seen as freaky shows just how far most people are sinking in the food trap and just how bad the situation has got. We are the only creatures on the planet that consider it odd or freakish if one of our own kind is *not* poisoning themselves on a regular basis, and we're the most intelligent – apparently.

It's ironic that the drug food and drinks industry spends literally billions of pounds every year advertising its wares, yet the biggest sales force they have actually pays them. Yes, it's the drug food addicts themselves – the very people who are hooked are the ones who do the biggest advertising for these organizations. The next time you are at a restaurant just listen to how the person who wants a dessert describes it; how they 'advertise' these drug foods to their friends. The words they use and their facial expressions and the ums and rrrr's would be worthy of any Saatchi & Saatchi advertising campaign. You see all they need is just one person to join them and they are happy, it means they can then 'indulge' (their word not mine). But if everyone says no, nine times out of ten they will also decide to skip dessert themselves. Why? For the simple reason already stated but worth repeating – when you are doing something which you instinctively know is pretty stupid you will feel less stupid if someone else is doing it with you. If they do get someone to join them with a dessert just listen to how they talk about it when it arrives. They constantly try to make you jealous, making all kinds of noises as they eat it, but what the hell is there to be jealous about? The image the menu gave and the words the drug food eater used to describe this 'delight' is always a far cry from the frozen lump of sugar and cow glue covered in theobromine-laced cocoa that has arrived at the table – oh with the squirt of 'cream in a can' on the side of course. And how do they feel *after* they have eaten it – not so happy then are they? Virtually every time they'll say 'Oh I wish I hadn't had that'. And even if they don't actually voice it, they will be thinking it. How do I know this for sure? Because not only have I treated thousands of people who all testify to this type of thinking, but more importantly because I've been there myself.

So watch those around you, unless you are aware of why they are saying the things they are saying they can pull you back

When people are on a diet, others around them don't mind as the person on the diet is almost doomed to misery and failure before they start. On top of that the dieter is constantly feeling deprived and voices how much they would love what the others are having. This simply confirms the false belief that people not on a diet are getting something special and the dieter who pines for, but declines, is the one missing out on some kind of benefit. This makes the non-dieters feel okay, in fact it makes them feel sorry for the dieter. However, because you are not going to be on a diet, not moping and will be actually pitying them for the poor drug food addicts they are, a part of their brain will resent you. Your change is affecting them because they would *ideally* love to be in your position but feel as though it's out of their reach. So if they can't get to where you are the next best thing is to try and tear you down.

So when you hear members of the food police banging on about what you eat or don't eat, please remember it's *only* because they feel insignificant around you. This leads them to justify their actions very loudly at the same time as bringing you down – it's simply a need to feel significant. You will get exactly the same reaction from 'The Gym Police' when you are regularly participating in the best exercise programme in the world – so be prepared.

HOW LONG HAS IT BEEN?

You will also get the 'how long has it been' gang. These people will say things like 'Well how long has it been? I wouldn't speak too soon it is, after all, early days yet'. These are the people who gauge your success by length of time and by your past 'attempts' to change. But what they won't know is you are not 'attempting' to do this, you have made a true decision and have *already* done it. And what the hell has time got to do with it? Does it really matter how long you've been free as long as you are free? What these people don't realize is that you are free from your old eating habits for LIFE. And that freedom started from day one. The last thing you'll be doing is counting the days. That is what dieting is all about: sitting indoors counting the days, waiting for the day you might actually be happy your decision, waiting for the day you can say to the world, 'I've done it. I don't need to eat that rubbish any more. I'm going to start living. I'm free'. But the point I want to hammer home is why wait? The truth is you can say it from day one. If you do not say it on day one then when are you going to say it?

You are free from the start so rejoice from the start

Did Nelson Mandela get this nonsense when he was released from prison? Did people say, 'I wouldn't celebrate yet Nelson, it's only been a week'? Length of time means nothing. It only means something while you are waiting for your release date, but once released – it's over at that moment. Nelson Mandela only counted the days he was *in* prison. Once you are free you are free. But you need to realize that the food police don't understand this concept and it often freaks them out. The truth is they don't want you to be eating healthily, moving your body regularly *and* being cheerful at the same time. Remember they don't mind you changing – providing you're miserable.

So just watch out and be aware of exactly why people do what they do. And don't forget that the same thing that got us all lured into the food trap in the first place is still out there – the advertising, brain-washing and conditioning. And the biggest advertising is done by the very people who are slap-bang in the food trap.

Am I saying that everyone will do this kind of thing? No. I am just pointing out that some people will behave in this way and that it will happen most during the first few weeks. This is why it is essential for you to know exactly why they are doing it. It is also essential for you to recognize certain physical and mental triggers, which, unless fully understood, could lead to a jump back to diet mentality. These triggers happen *automatically*, sending certain thoughts to your mind during the adjustment period. These can be caused by the 'bells' (cinema equals popcorn for example) or by the false physical hungers (drug food and drink hangovers). Such triggers are nothing to worry about, but you do need to know why they are happening so that you don't start to panic.

As I have repeatedly said, it's easy to make the change but your brain needs a little time to adjust to any new situation. So please – and this is a key ingredient of the ultimate health recipe – during the first couple of weeks it is essential to...

35

Give Your
Brain a Break

Your brain is the most ingenious computer in the world and yes it will adjust to *any* new situation, but please understand that as magnificent as your brain may be, it will take a little time to adjust fully to your new lifestyle.

ADJUSTING TO THE SWITCH

It's a bit like when you change your car. Sod's law the indicator switch seems to always be on the other side. What happens when you want to indicate on the first day of driving the new car? You put your windscreen wipers on. Why? Is it because you secretly wanted to wipe the windscreen? Is it a sign from the universe that you want your old car back? Is it your brain's way of telling you you don't deserve a new car? Of course it isn't – it's just your brain adjusting to the new situation. The first day you drive the new car, every time you take a corner you put the windscreen wipers on by mistake. Not sometimes – every single time. Do you get stressed, get massive insecurity attacks and say things to yourself like, 'Oh my God I'm never going to adjust to this, I need my old car back' ? NO OF COURSE YOU DON'T. All you do switch the indicators on and get on with driving in the direction you want to go. Even though you put the wipers on every single time that you want to indicate on the *first day*, you never think for one second that you won't adjust to it. This is because you are not *hoping* you are going to adjust – you *know for certain* that you will. This is why you don't go to bed the first night worrying about whether the same thing will happen the next day or every day for the rest of your life. All you think about is how wonderful it feels to be driving your new car. The second day you drive the car the amount of times you wipe instead of indicate is literally halved. The next day, it's halved again, then halved again and again and within no time at all you have fully adjusted to the new car. And exactly the same thing will happen with what you are achieving.

GIVE US A BELL

You may find that certain situations and feelings will make you automatically think about drug foods and drinks, for example when you enter a cinema and think of popcorn and cola. But just because you think of them it doesn't mean you still want them – it's just your *mental* windscreen wipers. Whenever you are in any situation where out of the blue you find certain drug foods and drinks pop into your head, all it means is that something, either a *false* mental hunger (a bell or trigger) or a *false* physical hunger (drug food and drink withdrawal), automatically made you *think* about them. But again, this doesn't mean that something has gone wrong with the way you are thinking – it's simply part of the adjustment. In fact it would be abnormal for these thoughts not to pop into your head every now and then.

It's like if you go on the same route to work every day for months or years. You become so 'conditioned' to the route that you can find yourself heading there even on your day off when you planned to go to a completely different place. The point I am making again is once you realize that you have headed in the wrong direction, do you go to work anyway simply because you're already half way there? NO WAY. You realize what's happening and do a sharp U-turn. And you will find yourself doing exactly the same thing in various situations when it comes to certain foods and drinks.

OFF YOUR TROLLEY

Another good example of this is the 'supermarket shopping route'. Anybody who regularly shops in the same supermarket will have one of these – a set route planned in your mind before you even enter the store. This is why supermarkets are forever changing things around; they know we have a set route that we stick to and they know we will automatically go to where things used to be not just once, but several times until we get used to their new position. The point is because you have been travelling on the same 'food' route for years it is perfectly normal, especially during the first three weeks, for your mind and body to automatically start heading in the direction of your old brand of food and drinks. If you find yourself doing this at times, just like the route to work analogy, don't panic – DO A SHARP U-TURN AND FEEL RELIEVED THAT YOU NO LONGER HAVE TO GO THERE.

There are loads of situations that can create automatic thoughts with regard to certain foods and drinks. Remember these are only thoughts. All kinds of things can trigger a thought, but a thought is just a thought. A thought holds no power over you other than the power you give it. We think of all kinds of things, but do we act on all our thoughts? NO – if we did we'd be arrested! Thinking about drug-like foods and drinks is *not* the problem – it's *what* you think that matters. John McCarthy was locked up for seven years in the Lebanon: did he think about the Lebanon when he was first released? Of course he did. In fact he probably thought about it more during the first few weeks than at any other time. The point is yes he did think about the Lebanon and yes he had to experience a period of adjustment after his release, but I can guarantee he loved the adjustment – no matter how strange it felt at first. And I can be certain that when Lebanon was in his thoughts he never thought, 'Oh I'd love to go back there for a treat'! His overriding thought was, 'Thank god I'm free'. That's exactly what I thought when I was first released from the food trap and it's precisely what I think now – *'Thank God I'm free'*.

TRY NOT TO THINK OF CHOCOLATE

Another mistake we tend to make when trying to kick certain foods and drinks is to try not to think about them. We even try to keep ourselves busy so that our minds are occupied with other thoughts. But does this work? NO. Once again this is diet recipe stuff and it has completely the opposite effect. You cannot try to *not* think about something – it's impossible. If I said to you please try not to think about Michael Jackson, what are you immediately thinking about? Michael Jackson. And exactly the same happens if you try not to think about something like chocolate. If you try not to think about anything you are bound to think about the very thing you are trying not to think about. The idea is *not* to avoid the thought, or try to think of something else, or worry that you are thinking it: the answer is to acknowledge it for what it is and jump for joy you don't have to act on it any more – that you are free. Remember, thinking about the drug foods and drinks that you have dumped from your life doesn't matter a jot – it's *what* you think that counts. In fact, in order to remain free for life, I want you to make a point of thinking about them. The people who forget about what these so-called foods really are tend to be the ones who get sucked back in again.

STARVING THE PARASITES

It's worth reminding ourselves that some of the 'mental windscreen wipers' (automatic thoughts) are directly caused by the physical drug-like food and drink parasites calling for their fix. Remember, what makes the food trap so ingenious is the way the industry has managed to create a false need in their consumers. Drug foods and drinks actually create additional feelings of emptiness (hunger) that seemingly are *only* instantly filled with more of the same. The more people consume, the bigger the emptiness they feel, the bigger the void, the more they try and fill it – this is the essence of the food trap and should be crystal clear by now. People stay mentally locked in the food trap because drug food and drinks appear to fill the very emptiness they helped to create.

Under normal circumstances it is quite natural to feel insecure, get stressed and panic if you are hungry and believe you can't end it for whatever reason. We were specifically designed to feel insecure and fearful. Hunger is, after all, nature's way of saying GO AND EAT. A slight *physical* hunger can blow into full blown *mental* panic if you think you will be deprived of food. However, all you need to remember is that as long as you are following the Juice Master's recipe for success, you will be feeding every cell in your body, so there is nothing to panic about. If you do feel any hunger between your meal times, you can be assured these are simply the *false* hungers and they will soon be gone for good. They cannot be fed with natural food and they cannot go away with drug foods, for they are the cause. The only way to get rid of them is to recognize them for what they are and enjoy starving them to death.

If you do ever get a thought that makes you believe that it is YOU that wants these nightmare foods during the adjustment period, remember why you are reading this book, why you are making the change, why you have made the decision to get busy living. It's not you who wants them, *you* want to be free. So change the thought from 'I want' to 'IT wants'. 'It' being whatever drug food or drink parasite is daring to rear its ugly head in a desperate attempt to survive.

In fact if you get any thought at all, whether it is a parasite demanding that you feed it, an empty feeling or a mental trigger or 'bell' during the first couple of weeks do yourself a favour – blame it *all* on the parasites and experience how wonderful it feels to say, 'STUFF YOU, I'M FREE'. Experience how brilliant it feels to know that each time you don't feed the blighters, each time you let them starve, you are one step closer to ultimate freedom and one day closer to the land of the slim and healthy for life.

Am I saying that you are going to be pestered with the parasites calling all the time? No. On the contrary, with the help of the fastest food in the west and the good wholesome solid foods that you will be eating, most of the time you won't be aware of anything at all. Of course the proof of the pudding is in the eating, but the majority of people are so juiced they don't notice a thing.

WELL DONE – YOU'VE PASSED

Understanding this book is a bit like passing your driving test. When you first pass your test the liberating feeling is amazing. In fact I remember waving my pink slip at people at bus stops on the way back from the test centre with the biggest grin in the world on my face and yelling, 'Yes, Yes, Yes!'. I wasn't simply happy when I passed my driving test – I WAS EUPHORIC. But just like every single person in the world who passes their driving test – I couldn't actually drive. Now you may think that my examiner made a mistake by passing me, but the truth is nobody can drive when they *first* pass their test – they learn to drive in the few weeks *after* they pass. The first week you're still *thinking* about clutch control, looking in your mirrors etc. If someone talks to you whilst you are driving you tell them to shut up because you need to concentrate. But in no time at all you're talking, changing the radio station and driving at the same time without even thinking about any of the mechanics – it becomes automatic. Each and every day you become a better driver. Your brain soon adjusts and something you once thought difficult becomes automatic. And exactly the same goes for the change you are making here. In no time at all your new regime of juicing, eating, breathing and doing the best exercise programme in the world becomes as automatic as brushing your teeth. The exciting news is that if you have already made the decision it means that you've already passed and you are already mentally free. This means the mental juice part of the recipe is taken care of. All that's left are the practicalities on the physical front. Let's start then with the most important meal of the day. Yes you finally have full permission to...

36

Breakfast Like a King

When I say breakfast like a king I DON'T MEAN HENRY VIII. He's hardly the best *roll* model now is he? No, I mean it's time to treat the inside of your body like royalty and furnish it with the finest breakfast in the land. It's time to give as much attention to cleaning the inside of your body in the morning as you do the outside.

WASHING WITH GLUE AND PASTE

You wouldn't dream of leaving the house in the morning without first cleaning your teeth and having a shower would you? In fact many people spend hours every day cleaning, toning and moisturizing the *outside* of their body, yet wouldn't dream of cleaning the inside. All the 're-vitalizing' external creams in the world mean nothing – vitality comes from *within*. How clean would you be if every morning you washed yourself, not with water, but with cream cheese, white paste and coffee? How groggy would you feel if your all-over shower gel was made of cow glue and maple syrup? So how on earth is your body ever expected to cleanse itself if that's what it wakes up to? Well IT SIMPLY CAN'T.

Of all the things I teach on the physical side, getting the right start in the morning is one of the single most important things you can do to restore health and vitality and aid weight loss. What you put in your system in the first few hours of waking is a *very, very* important part of the ultimate health recipe. Here's why. When you are sleeping the body repairs itself and *eliminates* toxins much faster than when you're awake. When you wake, your body is still in the process of eliminating waste from your system. The body uses whatever outlets are available to chuck the rubbish out. This is why your hair sticks together, you sweat, you have sleep in your eyes, your armpits stink, your mouth feels like the inside of Ghandi's flip flop, your breath is straight from Satan's bottom – and you need to head straight for the loo.

All of these signs are in a way good, as they mean the body is doing its utmost to keep you well and alive. It means it's cleaning out the rubbish, and for the first 4–5 hours after you wake it wants to *continue* eliminating waste. I do realize that the body is always eliminating waste to varying degrees, but this is the time when it's most obvious and it's the best time for you to aid the process. The last thing the body needs is more toxins coming in when it's still trying to throw yesterday's out. It can certainly do without having to use vital nerve energy to digest and process junk or drug foods when it's trying to use the energy to rid itself of toxic waste. The body needs to cleanse and the morning is an ideal time to help the process. At the same time you'll be kick-starting your system and feeding vital nutrients to your cells.

THE JUICE MASTER'S FAST FOOD BREAKFAST
First course
WATER

All life on this planet simply would not exist without this stuff – it is an absolute must. We are dehydrating all the time and most of the time we aren't even aware of it. We lose about two litres a day; if you move your body a lot or it's a hot day, you lose even more. It is essential to have clear, nothing-added, cleansing, hydrating liquid entering your system several times a day – *especially* first thing in the morning. During the night there is no question that as the body detoxifies it loses water in the process, usually through sweat. This means that, whether you actually feel it or not, you are going to always wake up slightly dehydrated. So I strongly advise that the first thing to enter your system should be a body-cleansing glass of clear water.

Second course
OXYGEN

Yes oxygen. You won't see that on many breakfast menus that's for sure. Now before you start thinking this is turning into the 'Fresh Air' diet, let me put your mind at rest. The idea behind the Juice Master fast food breakfast is to *feed* your body and cells with everything they need to satisfy your hunger for a good few hours, *without* interfering with the process of elimination. When your cells are hungry the first thing they need is oxygen. Oxygen feeds *every* single cell in your body and without it, you die. Now you may think that we breathe anyway and must get enough oxygen, so why not just skip the second course and get straight to the main course? Because although you obviously get enough oxygen to survive when you breathe normally, it's not enough for a *good* feed and it's certainly not enough to truly cleanse your lymph system. Our ancestors certainly wouldn't have had this problem. They had to move for survival purposes and thus cleansed their lymph systems automatically. However, we are not active enough and most of us do not breathe in a way that aids the lymph system. It has been medically proven that the single most effective way to clean your lymph system is by deep breathing. So with that in mind, relish your second course and treat yourself to a good blast of oxygen first thing every morning. You will be amazed at what 10–20 deep long breaths three times daily can do for you. Yoga is simply amazing for this, but if that's not your bag, you can either just do some deep breathing (make sure your stomach comes out when you breathe in) or you can get up and do the best exercise programme in the world.

There's nothing like a good bounce in the morning

Personally I vary it. Sometimes I do some deep breathing or 15–30 minutes yoga, and sometimes I can't wait to do the best exercise programme in the world – which varies depending on the weather or what I'm into at the time. At the moment I don't think you can beat a good bounce first thing (and yes I do mean on my trampoline). This might be your idea of living hell, if it is DON'T DO IT. Just make certain you blast your cells with some oxygen in a way that works for you. After you've given yourself a good dose of life-giving, body-cleansing, lymphomaniac oxygen it's on to the next course.

Main course
THE FASTEST FOOD IN THE WEST *or*
THE ULTIMATE FAT-BUSTING HEALTH PILL
(*or* A COMBINATION OF THE TWO)

And my what a choice you now have. When I first made the change I thought just having fruit in the morning wouldn't give me much variety, but I couldn't have been more wrong. There are just so many different kinds of mouthwatering fruits from around the world with so many different, tantalizing flavours and each one bursting with such vibrant colour. It certainly beats the hell out of sugar carbs covered in cow glue every morning that's for sure. And come to think of it, why on earth did I think I'd be missing out on variety? There wasn't exactly much variety in cereal with milk and toast every morning, was there?

You have an unbelievable variety of fruits, juices and smoothies (whole soft fruits mixed with fruit juice in a blender) available to break your fast every morning of the year in the fastest possible way. There are over ten different types of melon, each with a unique taste and colour – and that's just one fruit. There is so much you can do with fruit once you get going. I must admit when I first started I was fruit and vegetable illiterate (if there is such a thing). I didn't have the faintest idea of the amazing things you can do with it once you expand your mind and use a little imagination. You can, of course, simply eat the fruits as they are – a big bowl of fresh strawberries, chunks of mango, kiwi fruit, pineapple slices, grated coconut etc. looks and tastes truly amazing. But if you want to free up even more energy for weight loss, flush your system, have loads more variety available to you and be certain you are getting your daily requirements of *live* nutrients in the fastest way possible then you will need two vital pieces of equipment.

A JUICING MACHINE AND A BLENDER

These two machines will be the best investments in terms of health you will ever make in your life (I'll recommend some models later). The only reason I manage to get enough *live* nutrients, especially of the raw vegetable kind, flowing through my system is because I juice – every single day. It is the fastest food in the west and the benefits are unbelievable. Plus you can do so much more with your fast food breakfast once you have these two life-saving machines.

You can put frozen blackberries, fresh strawberries and pineapple chunks in the blender, add a little water and ice and boom you have a glass of pure *live* nutrition which looks and tastes incredible. How about some almonds, frozen banana, frozen chunks of mango, frozen berries, couple of ice cubes, blend and eat like a ice cream – great for summer. If you have kids they just love the whole process of juicing – they're fascinated by it so it's easy to get them to drink it too. You can wake up to a Berry Maguire, a Caribbean Dream or get yourself moving (literally) with The Jack 'Sun' Five (see recipes on pages 288 to 296).

There are so many tantalizing ways to break your fast with a JM fast food breakfast that it would take you another year to finish the book if I included them. I have included some recipes at the back of the book to get you started, but if you want different combinations to meet what *you* fancy – just experiment. Remember there are no set rules, have it *your* way. If you would prefer more recipes and an in-depth, light-hearted, guide to juicing, blending and how to set up a Juice Master kitchen then get hold of a copy of *The Juice Master's Ultimate Fast Food* book or video or come to a seminar/workshop to see juicing in action (for info on both see page 309).

One thing you must remember when it comes to juicing is that once the fruits have been exposed to air they will begin to lose some of their life force. Ever taken a bite of an apple and left it out? It goes brown. This is called oxidization – or *starting to die* as I call it. After it has been left for a couple of hours it's as good as enzyme empty – or dead. Therefore it is *essential* that you drink your juice as soon as you've made it (or within the first 1–2 hours – the sooner the better). If, for whatever reason, it has been left for a good few hours, don't throw it away as it still is a good source of carbs and water and still makes a tasty drink – just don't forget to shake it.

A tip for keeping your juice longer is to get an empty flask and put it in the freezer with the lid off. Next morning, make your juice, pour into the flask and seal with the lid *immediately*. That way the ice cold temperature and sealed unit of the flask will keep your juice for much longer. This is good for making vegetable juice in the morning to have with lunch. It does also depend on the machine you use – there is one which extracts the juice in such a way that enables you keep it in your fridge for three days (see page 286). Another tip is to add lemon juice to your juice (fruit or veg) to slow down deterioration. Have you noticed how quickly an avocado goes black when it's exposed to air? And how it stays fresher for longer with a touch of lemon juice? Nature – you just can't beat it.

So how much can I have Mr Juice Master?

Well you can *eat* as much fruit as you like during the first 5–6 hours of waking, especially during the adjustment period. You will find that after a short while, as your false hungers die and you are feeding your body once again with what it really needs, you just won't need that much and your hunger will be satisfied for longer. With fruit *juice*, I would advise no more than 1 pint maximum, drunk over a 1–2 hour period in the mornings. I would also advise that you always add ice and some water to prevent the juice being too concentrated. Although fruit is a good source of natural sugar, even too much of a good thing can be bad. Bear in mind that we wouldn't normally eat six oranges, a banana, half a pound of strawberries, half a pineapple etc. all in one go and too much of even the good sugars *can* cause your body to over-secrete insulin – which is the last thing you want. This is why when you do make a smoothie you should add a small amount of ice and water and *take your time* with it. A smoothie or juice is like a meal in itself and as such should be 'chewed'. What I mean is, swill it around in your mouth first, don't just gulp down a pint in one minute flat! If you do that you *will* have problems.

If you are diabetic, suffer from candida, have athlete's foot, thrush or are already suffering from low blood sugar and/or have a weight problem, then make your fruit juice with about *half* mineral water, that way there is no danger of loading your bloodstream with too much natural sugar. Also, have smoothies, rather than just juice, as whole fruits with fibre slow down the rate at which sugars are released into the bloodstream. Another good tip is to add some nuts, such as *natural* almonds, to the blender, as again it helps prevent a rapid absorption of concentrated fruit sugars into the bloodstream. Better still, and for best results, if you're trying to lose weight, during the first month, make a point of –

Eating your fruit and drinking your veggies!

Clearly that doesn't mean don't *eat* veggies (tuck into those babies whenever you wish!), it just means when it comes to raw 'live' liquid gold juice – go for JM's veggies and eat the mouth-watering array of fruits that are always on offer. This doesn't mean you can never have beautiful fruit juices or smoothies, it just means if you suffer from any of the above-mentioned problems, the pancreas is going to need a few weeks repair time, essential if you have a weight problem. If you do have fruit during the first month, as well you might due to the fact that they're scrummy, please *always* make a point of following the guide-lines I've just given. As you are changing your brand from the start, and given for the first month concentrated fruit juices could be a weight-loss stopper, why not kick start your day – The Juice Master way!

'A vegetable juice, made in the right way, first thing in the morning is pure health heaven. Using the fruit apple here as part of the JM veggie base is fine, as apple juice is very fructose based, meaning no excess sugar problems. Once again, though, take your time with it – it is a meal. There is, however, no need to add water or ice. If you keep your vegetables in the fridge and then juice them, you instantly have a cool veg juice. Most people, however, opt for the fruit versions in the morning (using my guidelines) to *break* their *fast* in the mornings, as I used to, and occasionally still do, but the sooner you give your taste buds a good training and get on to the pure liquid magic that is veggie juice, the better. Drinking rich, creamy, sweet-tasting veggie juice in the morning and *eating* some organic apples to go along with it will have you radiant, slim and healthy in no time. Again, when you eat fruit (except hybrid mass-produced bananas) there is no danger of loading the bloodstream with too much sugar, it's only if you drink loads of it undiluted and very fast that you can possibly experience problems. You really have to go some for fruit to cause you problems so follow my guidelines and enjoy heaven in a glass. If you are diabetic and in doubt please *always* consult your doctor first.'

I don't usually have breakfast anyway so is it okay just to skip the juice, smoothie or fruit?
NO! NO! NO! NO! NO! NO! NO! NO! NO! NO! NO! NO! NO! NO! NO! NO! NO! NO!

Although your body is cleaning house first thing in the morning don't skip the JM's fast food breakfast. It is VERY important to kick-start your system and feed your cells. It is also vital you keep your sugar levels in check and employ your enzyme workforce. If you don't, you will reach the stage where you get uncomfortably hungry and this can cause your parasites to rear their ugly heads and convince you that only way to solve this hunger is by feeding them and giving yourself a quick fix. So nuke the little suckers with a good blast of water, oxygen and the fastest food in the west before they even get a look in. Starting your day right also has a wonderful knock-on effect to everything you do for the rest of your day.

So from this point on really treat yourself by breaking your fast with a JM fast food breakfast. It's specifically designed to really feed the body, help with the cleansing process and get you to the land of the slim and healthy. Expand your mind, look at *all* the different fruits available to you, invest in a juicer and a blender, use your imagination and give yourself permission to truly breakfast like a king. Well, that's breakfast well and truly taken care of, now...

37

Let's Do Lunch

So what can I have for lunch?

Many times when you feel hungry, the body is actually crying out for water. You will find that you eat less food at meal times if you have a good glass of water first. First course, therefore – water! I cannot stress enough the importance of this incredible body-cleansing substance. So what's for lunch then? Remember, there are no rules any more – *you* are in charge of what you eat from now on. So with that in mind, what do you feel like? If you want some chicken, fish or – if you really must – steak, then have it. Just make sure you have a *large* water-rich salad with it. High water content, live-nutrient-packed meals are the key to being healthy and slim. They help to flush the system, feed the body and supply a much-needed digestive enzyme workforce to help break down, use and dispose of whatever junk (not drug) food you are eating at the same time. If you are the same as I was and not used to eating salads at all, bear in mind that for you to have *lifetime* success you are changing your brand and, as such, you are putting yourself in the 'taste gym' for a few weeks. In no time at all you will learn to love the foods you once called 'rabbit food'. This doesn't mean you have to train yourself to like *all* vegetables – after all I still don't think we were ever meant to like Brussels sprouts! It just means find what works for you. I hate cooked cabbage and I have no desire to eat cabbage leaves, but I often grate red cabbage and sprinkle it over my JM salad (see pages 294–5). In order for me to enjoy a salad it's got to consist of a hell of a lot more than a bowl full of iceberg lettuce, a couple of sad-looking tomatoes and some soggy cucumber – it's amazing what you can do with a little imagination.

So for lunch it really just comes down to following a couple of guidelines – 'live' nutrient-packed water-rich foods, eaten either by themselves, with easy to digest proteins (tuna, sardines, etc.), or with 'whole', close as to original carbs as you can get. Then it's simply a case of figuring out what YOU want from the thousands of choices available to you every day. How about a big tuna salad; chicken with stir-fried veg; the JM daytime snack – lightly toasted rye-bread spread with creamy avocado, some sardines and lovely lemon juice over the top to add some zest; avocado, tomato, lemon juice salad sandwich in wholemeal bread? What about a nice piece of fish with steamed broccoli, mangetout, baby corn on the cob and a *few* new potatoes? How about some home-made avocado dip (avocados in blender with lemon juice and tomatoes) with a bright beautiful JM salad and a couple of warm wholemeal pitta breads? Chicken salad with a glass of pure life-giving, nutrient-packed vegetable juice?

All of these feed the body, help to flush the system and are correctly combined. Again, I cannot list everything that meets with the JM's ultimate health recipe because I'd be here for a year. The point is you are *not* going to starve from now on. As I have mentioned over and over again, you are simply changing the way you think in order to be happy about changing your brand – and by changing your brand you'll *stop* starving yourself.

JUICE WITH LUNCH

If you are in the mood and would love a super kick-start to your journey to Mauritius then juice once again is the key. A big main course salad with a pint of vegetable juice is literally sunshine for your body. I have about a pint of freshly-made vegetable juice (usually the Dy'Sun' blended with half a small avocado) at least 3–4 days a week for lunch. I find that even if I'm very hungry the live nutrients in the juice and the good fats and proteins from the avocado more than satisfy my hunger within 15–20 minutes. If I get hungry again a bit later I have some fruit. Many people who have tried juicing have a *small* glass every other day. As far as I'm concerned the more enzymes the better. We have a very depleted account, so the more deposits of life force, the more life we are going to get and the better the results. This doesn't mean flood your body with vegetable juice until you feel uncomfortable – it just means if you are going to make it and it's all you're having then have a good pint of the stuff.

Vegetable juice is *very* important to this programme; drink one pint a day – preferably as a meal – and the difference to the way you feel will be quite simply unbelievable. Without veg juice the chances are you just won't get the amount of nutrients you need – so get juicing those veg.

Another excellent option is to continue with fruit and veg all through the day. I often do this and I know many of my clients use this as a tool 3–4 days a week. Having natural foods during the day, whether it's just fruit, or salads, or juices, has several massive advantages.

1 You are guaranteed to be feeding your body at least 60–70 per cent worth of high water content, natural nutrient-packed foods. The average person has 0–5 per cent.
2 You will be flushing your system for at least 16 hours a day.
3 You don't even have to think about timing and combining as all fruit and veg mix well with each other.
4 It makes you feel light, clear-headed and mentally and physically vibrant.
5 Your evening meal tastes amazing.

The fact is if you get the day right, your body will be so juiced with nutrients that it can virtually deal with anything you throw at it for dinner. If I know I'm going to a dinner party I always have a pure fruit, salad, veg and smoothie day. That way even if all that's there are foods that contain *no* live nutrients, like at a barbecue for example, my body can easily deal with it and I can enjoy as much as I like without worrying.

But what do I do if I find myself in a McDonalds at lunch-time? Get out!

I do realize that there are many people who 'do lunch' every day, so making a juice or taking one to work may prove tricky. The good news is that there are many excellent new-style cafes (not the greasy spoons) that offer brilliant salads and juices. But as with all of this be flexible, if you are doing lunch and you want it, then have some fish or chicken or whatever you like. The all-day natural food is, like combining, just a tool you can use whenever you feel it appropriate.
I often skip lunch and if I don't eat I'm better off on the weight-loss front aren't I?
NO! NO! NO! NO! NO! NO! NO! NO! NO! NO! NO! NO! NO! NO! NO! NO! NO! NO!

I cannot stress enough just how important it is to keep your blood sugar levels in check. It takes *energy* and live nutrients to lose weight, and fruit, veg, salads and their juices *all* contain the enzymes needed to balance the body, repair it and shift excess waste (fat). And, once again, if you let your sugar levels get too low it can cause you to become uncomfortably hungry and at times like that you really do reach for anything. So even if you don't feel like much, have some fruit, or if you find fruit, for whatever reason, isn't cutting the hunger mustard, then have some tuna-mayo or a slice of toasted rye bread with some creamy avocado and some sun-blush tomatoes (yes, I feel hungry now too!). The point is – have something!

Now after work and before we do dinner don't miss the chance to...

38

Go and Play

Early evening is the ideal time to go and play, whether it's going to the gym or kicking a ball around the park. As always do the best exercise programme in the world for you. If you are tired and feel hungry after work, do an aerobics class, or dance, or walk, or do some yoga, or whatever, instead of just going home, slumping on the settee and eating. If you have kids, play some basketball or have a game of rounders – whatever inspires and works for you. This may all sound a bit daunting for some at this stage, but in no time you will end up feeling deprived if you *don't* do it. You will find that what your body was really hungry for was *oxygen* and the main reason for the tiredness was a clogged lymph system, caused by inactivity. I often find that if I'm hungry and tired after work and do an aerobics class, or play some tennis, badminton, football or whatever I am nowhere near as tired or hungry as I was before.

There is also nothing quite like the feeling of total relaxation after exercise. Many gyms have steams rooms and saunas – sure beats the pub to unwind, and it's often more sociable too. You can then look forward to sitting down to the pleasure of satisfying a genuine appetite – guilt free of course.

So what wonderful food can you look forward to at the end of a fulfilling day? Well let's find out...

39

What's For Dinner?

Once again – WHAT DO YOU WANT? Hot whitebait on a bed of nutrient-packed salad? Some whole-grain pasta with fresh basil and pesto sauce? Some soup, with a wholemeal bread roll and organic butter, followed by rice and stir-fried veg? A large plate of organic chicken with steamed veg and salad? A large main course avocado salad, some warm wholemeal pitta bread and a small side order of chips (yes chips!). Remember, if you are genuinely physically hungry the body will digest just about anything, so if you are out having a meal and you want a few chips – have them. If you want to go out for a curry then go. This is not a diet – it's freedom from dieting and it's freedom from the food trap. So feel free to eat whatever takes your fancy, just dump the white refined trash, the majority of the wrong kinds of fats and supply your body with as much high water content, nutrient-packed food as possible at *every* meal. The idea is to starve the false hungers, genuinely feed the body, and change your brand – you are now in charge. The choices are almost infinite – experiment and use your imagination, *just make certain that 70–80 per cent of what goes in your mouth every day is high water content, nutrient-packed **fast** foods and drinks.*

Your new brand is mainly nature's fast food but that doesn't mean it's going to run away!

Big tip when it comes to eating, TAKE YOUR TIME OVER FOOD – that way you really get to enjoy it. I had problems for years because I thought I couldn't be without the wonderful pleasures of food, yet I often missed them. I didn't savour flavours, I often just shovelled it in – always mentally on the next fork-full whilst my mouth was full from the previous one. It was as if I just wanted to get it down my throat as quickly as possible so I could get to the next mouthful. In a way I would miss the meal and the pleasure – it was gone before I knew it, the only lasting reminder being a bloated stomach. If you want to get more pleasure from food than you ever have had, then train yourself to take your time over what you eat. Really savour the many flavours and make a point of chewing it thoroughly as *digestion starts in the mouth*. Eating too quickly can cause you to overeat – even on the good stuff. It takes a bit of time for your body to feel satisfied. If you eat very quickly, without really chewing your food, you can easily end up feeling bloated. Too much food of any kind at once can be too much of a burden for the stomach. So if you really want to get maximum pleasure from your eating time, eat slowly and enjoy.

JUICE WITH DINNER

To ensure you are getting an abundance of live nutrients, it's a good idea to have a glass of freshly-made vegetable juice with your evening meal – that way even if your main course is lacking in nutrients for whatever reason you are still getting them. As I've said, if you really can't eat a good quantity of vegetables at first while you're training your taste buds – then drink them. If you do have juice with your meal, treat the juice as part of the meal and sip it as you would wine. In fact a carrot, apple, spinach, celery and beetroot juice looks just like red wine when poured into a cold wine glass. It may sound, well, awful to many, but it's creamy and tastes wonderful – don't knock it till you've tried it. Talking of wine, if you still want a *couple* of glasses of wine with your evening meal a couple of times a week it's really not going to make or break your success – so feel free.

Some people choose to have their main meal around 4pm and then only have fruit and juices till bedtime – those who do have incredible success. This particular way of doing things doesn't fit with me when I'm in the UK, but it's whatever *you* want to do and whatever works for you and your lifestyle. One thing though, make sure that you eat your evening meal at least three hours before you go to sleep. I know this is difficult sometimes when you are forced to dine late but do it whenever possible. When you sleep your metabolism slows down massively and it is important that your stomach is empty, so that you can fully rest while you sleep. If you feel hungry before bedtime have some fruit. One of the single most effective tools for weight loss has to be the 6pm carb boycott. With this you really don't need to know the science, all you need to know is – IT WORKS! If you make it a rule, for at least five days a week *every* week, to have a protein-rich meal (fish, chicken, avocado, olives, veggies, etc.) for dinner and leave out *all* man-made carbs (bread, pasta, rice and even potatoes) after 6pm, you will see an amazing difference to your shape in no time at all. Again, it's what works for you, but I know several people who have adopted the Slim 4 Life lifestyle and made it a rule not to have man-made carbs after 6pm, and boy, oh boy, the results are simply incredible. I want to make this point cristal clear – so you can't say you didn't know – when people have juice in the morning, *whole* carbs in the day and a protein-rich dinner, the results are truly amazing in *every* case! Even now I still do the 6pm carb boycott at least four days a week, for no other reason than it makes me feel good and I don't fancy gaining weight again! Trust me on this, if you are overweight, now that you're in the right frame of mind, why not dive straight in and adopt the 6pm carb boycott whenever you can – it will literally help to 'shape' your future life.

As you can see this is not rocket science and it's not a rigid, starve-yourself programme. In fact the choices are seemingly infinite. It's about living and being free. And in order to feel totally free and to make certain your success is for life you must...

40

Be Flexible

and let common sense prevail

In order for this mental and physical recipe to have lifelong results you must be flexible. Do not become evangelical about food and do not label yourself, as it puts too many unnecessary restrictions on you in times of genuine need. I am not a 'vegetarian' nor am I a 'vegan' or a 'fruitarian', and I'm certainly not a 'breatharian'. I am a human being who eats wonderful food when I'm feeling hungry. Although I haven't actually eaten meat in over four years, it doesn't mean that I never would. If there wasn't anything else available and I was really hungry, I would eat it. A few pieces of organic chicken are much better, health-wise, than a plate full of white refined pasta. Some people will choose to quit meat on other grounds; if so fine. But if you're considering quitting it on the grounds of health, remember that white meat is often a good option.

I did once label myself 'vegan' for over two years. I found myself not eating at times when I was genuinely hungry and felt deprived because of it. I felt deprived because I was, at times, being deprived – I should have eaten. If you are in an airport, it's often tricky to get something you want. The salads are often a waste of time (mainly iceberg lettuce and nothing else), the fruit looks like it's been there a month and everything else smells good. Remember, there will be times like these when you deviate from your new brand, the key is not to lose sleep over it or start saying stupid things like, 'Oh no I've blown it all now'. The key is to be free to do this. Just to eat the best choice available and enjoy ending a genuine hunger – you can always clean-up at the first possible opportunity. Once you understand it, it becomes almost impossible to 'blow it'.

When I went away to finish this book I found myself getting hungry at the airport. Now I'm not a big fan of packaged sandwiches because they tend to have awful bread and glue-like fillings. But I was hungry and I knew I wouldn't eat again for a long time, so I ended up with a wholemeal tuna salad sandwich, which I do realize is 'badly combined', but I did say be flexible and quit with the food police already! My system is so juiced now that a tuna salad sandwich once in a blue moon is hardly going to collapse it. So use your common sense, choose the best option available wherever you are and be flexible – it's vital for your sanity and freedom for life.

THE FLEXI BREAKFAST

I have either eaten fruit, or had a fruit smoothie or vegetable juice for breakfast virtually every day since I made the decision to get busy living some six years ago now – and I strongly believe it's been one of the major keys to the success I've had. However, there have been odd times when I've opted for what I call the 'flexi breakfast'. For example, I was in Israel a few years back and a group of us slept on an isolated beach for 3–4 days. One night we went out and placed a huge net in-between a couple of buoys to catch some fish. We woke at sunrise, went out a small boat and pulled in a net full of fish. Once back on the beach we lit the barbecue and all had fresh fish for breakfast – it was beautiful. The point is to be flexible so that you are free to join in at times like this.

For some people breakfast will never be breakfast without getting their teeth into something. If that's you, please 'be flexible' and eat the best option. I find a couple of slices of toasted rye bread usually does the trick for most – yes, with butter! But if you fancy a boiled egg and some cereal with soya milk every now and then, feel more than free to tuck in.

Getting your oats in the morning

Every now and then you may want something hot on a cold winter's morn. If so, jumbo oats are your best bet – made with either warm soya milk or water and topped with fresh fruits and perhaps a hot cup of herbal tea, or just lemon juice in hot water (a great cleanser). Oats are fairly easy for the body to deal with and in the morning you do have access to a lot of energy which has been built up overnight. As previously mentioned, you want to use this for elimination and don't want to waste it on digesting cooked food, but the *odd* hot breakfast isn't going to interfere with your success. To your surprise, after you are used to fresh smoothies in the morning and/or whole fruit, you will find that you just won't want or miss hot breakfasts. The juices simply taste too good and make you feel energized and light. Every now and then the smell of a fry-up does smell nice. People say, 'That means you still want it and you're using willpower not to have it'. No it doesn't – I love the smell of petrol but I don't use willpower not to drink the stuff!

If you do choose to have something other than a JM fast-food breakfast, make sure you have a fast-food lunch that day and wait until the evening before having any other concentrated food. You can, of course, eat fruit all day if you wish after your flexi breakfast. One tip though, I wouldn't have a flexi breakfast until you are fully used to your JM fast-food breakfast – the morning part really is that important.

WHEN IN ROME

Being flexible also allows for the 'when in Rome' way of living. It means that if you go to Jamaica and want to just know what Jerk Chicken tastes like – you are free to do so. If you are in Tunisia and are curious about curried goat – you are free to tuck in. If you are in France and want some snails – go for it. If you're in China and you want some dog – maybe not! You haven't *always* got to apply the 'when in Rome' principle and when it comes to places like China I don't blame you for not, but it means if you do want to try the food of a particular country – YOU ARE TOTALLY FREE TO DO SO. This is why I don't label myself veggie or vegan and this is why I advise you don't either. It is also why, although I haven't eaten meat for some years now, I am not saying I *never* would again. So if the food police see me eating Jerk Chicken in Jamaica – don't come shouting.

So as long as you're not evangelical about food, you *take action* and follow *all* of the ultimate mental and physical health recipe, you free yourself from things like 'people phobia' and really start to suck the juice from life, then you will have what few do – total freedom from the food trap and a daily quality of life many simply dream of. I don't know what your story is or just how deep you've sunk into the food trap, but one thing's for sure – as from *now* it all begins to change.

Don't forget to enjoy the journey as much as arriving there and don't forget when you wake up each morning you have a choice: you can either get busy living or you get busy dying – as always it's up to you. Remember, there is no in-between – you are either sucking the juice from life or it's sucking the juice from you. With that in mind it's worth reminding yourself as you go to bed each night that you are finally on your way to the land of the slim and healthy – Mauritius. And when you open your eyes in the morning, get excited because in case no one has told you up until now, or in case you forgot...

41

You've Got a Ticket to the Big Game

**Yes indeedy – you have a big ticket to the big game!
So what ya gonna do with it?**

Have you noticed how children can't sleep on Christmas eve and how they are up at 4am asking if it's time to open the presents yet? Ever noticed how excited they are, how alive they are, the look of joyous anticipation that lights up their face? It's a very different story though when they have to get up for school. If you *have* to get up to do something which doesn't inspire you it's tricky lifting your head off the pillow. Yet if you're going on a once-in-a-lifetime holiday you're up like a shot! Well it's time to start getting up like a shot because you have a unique ticket to the big game. The only question is – *what are you going to do with it?*

I see it like this. Life is a holiday lasting roughly a hundred or so years. Now even on holiday you have good and bad days. The problem is many people believe they've got a lousy deal from their holiday firm and have been landed with the holiday from hell. What they fail to realize is that...

WE ARE OUR OWN TOUR OPERATORS

This means it's up to *us*, not 'them' to design the holiday of our dreams. *We* get the unique chance each and every day to write the script and play in the big game. You can be sure of one thing, if we don't write our own script, if we don't take charge of our own game, there are millions of people who are paid massive amounts of money to write the script and play the game for us. You have seen this with the food companies and the way they use advertising and chemicals to write your script for you and use your big ticket for their financial gain. The idea is to take charge of your life each and every day, because we only get one ticket and each day really is a *once* in a lifetime day.

'Life is what happens while you're busy making other plans'

John Lennon

We get about 85–100 Christmases', and that's if we look after our incredible machine. We get the same amount of birthdays, and the same amount of TODAYs. Once it's gone – IT'S GONE. You can't just 'do it later' , because in terms of today, there is no later – today only happens once. It's a one shot deal. This is why feeling physically and mentally vibrant is so important – it gives us a chance to really play the game. And there is no question that you play a much better game when you feel light, clear-headed and alive. Each day is unique, each day is part of the game and as long as the clock's ticking (your heart) – you're still in it.

We are all so busy working for tomorrow that we so often fail to appreciate or capture today, this moment, this second of our lives. As John Lennon wrote, 'Life is what happens while you're busy making other plans' – so don't miss it while you are busy making plans.

CARPE DIEM (SEIZE THE DAY)

Many people play the 'I'll be happy when...' game. And it's one you never win. I'll be happy *when* I earn this amount of money. I'll be happy *when* I get this new car. I'll be happy *when* I reach the top etc. This amounts to always living in the future, thus missing today – right now. I still play the 'I'll be happy when...' game, but I've changed the rules slightly. Now I'll be happy when...ever I feel like it! So don't say, I'll be happy *when* the weight comes off or I'll be happy when I'm healthy. If you do that you've missed the point and all you'll be really saying is, 'I'll be miserable until I've lost the weight' – but why? There's no need, that's the 'Diet Recipe' remember? The whole point, the whole message of this book is to make you see the process is easy when you're *not* sitting around waiting for something to happen and it's the process that's the good part. It's about enjoying the journey, not just getting there so –

Don't be a weight watcher

If you are overweight and you follow the recipe then the excess weight will come off –but not *tomorrow*. You don't need to be Sherlock Holmes to figure out that it takes time to lose weight. So don't sit there staring at it each day to see if there's a difference and don't jump on the scales every day or week to see if you've dropped a few pounds. In fact – THROW YOUR SCALES AWAY and really set yourself free. It is not normal to weigh yourself, it only appears normal because so many people do it. If you watch a kettle it seems to take forever to boil and if you watch your weight the fat never seems to budge – so get on with living your life and delegate the process of fat removal to your body, it will do it for you. Just give it time.

THE FINEST DRUG TO BOOST YOUR GAME

One of the biggest joys of no longer using drug foods or drinks to try and change my emotional state, was the realization that we already own and have 24-hour access to the finest drug in the world in its purest form and IT'S FREE OF CHARGE. It's also the only drug that *genuinely* boosts every area of your game: pure adrenalin – life force. It's the buzz and excitement of being and feeling alive: growing each and every day, actually facing and meeting new challenges instead of first turning to, or trying to hide behind, food or drugs; the confidence to go out and truly live, regardless of what people may or may not think; the courage to *just do it*, whatever *it* is in that moment.

Drug foods and drinks are not only dead nutritionally, they also kill your life force. They *slowly* make you die inside. The problem is, because it happens so slowly, so gradually, most people don't notice it happening. People who are stuck in the food trap, hooked on drug-like foods and drinks, have no idea just how much these poisons are affecting so many areas of their lives. They look around and see they are pretty much the same as most other people and that is my point –

You don't want to be the same as over 90 per cent of the population

Most people are missing out on the juice of life. *Most* people simply survive but don't live. *Most* people have stress and not challenges. *Most* people are fat. *Most* people are ill. *Most* people end up in hospital or a nursing home. *Most* people are hooked. *Most* people are being controlled. *Most* people are people phobic. *Most* people reach for a food to try and change the way they feel, and *most* people don't realize they have a ticket to the big game. You really don't want to be like *most* people and from now on you don't have to be.

Now that you are breaking free you will always feel more physically and mentally vibrant and much more alive. This gives you the resources to tap into a quality of life you had forgotten existed. So enjoy the journey, don't forget about today, furnish your body with the finest nutrition available and get busy living. But beware though, no matter how long it has been since you made the change, the facts about drug foods and drinks NEVER change, but their relevance to you will. So in order to make sure your freedom is for life and you don't start to look back with rose-tinted glasses it is *essential* to add the final ingredient to the Ultimate Health Recipe...

42

Re-tune,
Re-tune and
Re-tune

Be aware that the same thing that lured you into consuming these nightmare foods is still out there. The advertising, the brainwashing, the bells and the peer pressure are all still out there, so be alert and flood you mind with mental juice on a regular basis – in other words, re-tune.

This is a very important ingredient of being slim, healthy and vibrant *for life*. In fact this ingredient is the one which makes the difference between slim for *life* and slim and for a *month* – so understand it and use it. If you miss just one ingredient from any kind of recipe you will get a different end result, and the same applies to the JM Ultimate Health Recipe. Everything I have put in this book is here for a reason and this re-tuning thing is a very important element of staying free.

There are many people who make changes in life, but so often they are short lived. They succeed for a while only to find themselves creeping back to their old ways. They claim to have been doing fine for a year but then they just found themselves one day craving other foods. Here's my point – it didn't happen just ONE DAY. Each and every day we are bombarded with thousands of images for drug foods and drinks. Each and every day we are surrounded by numerous poor souls who are still rooted in the food trap, each one trying to convince us that *we* are the ones missing out. Then there are many people who are specifically paid huge sums of money to change the way we think, to get us hooked on their brand of 'food'. The good news is that once you have removed the brainwashing and seen the truth, it takes a lot of images and a long time before your brain gets sucked back in to believing any of it. The point is you don't want to *ever* get sucked back in again, you want to keep this stuff crystal clear in your mind. As you will by now have realized, as long as you *think* the right way, it's easy to make the change – it's also very *easy* for that change to stick. This final ingredient is not in any way a penance or hard work. All you have to do is simply *re-tune* once in a while.

IF YOUR BRAIN REMAINS CLEAR OF THE RUBBISH THEN YOU *STAY* SLIM, HEALTHY AND FREE FOR LIFE

This is why it is essential for you to keep hold of this book – it is a re-tuning tool. If you lend it out, like a CD, you can be almost guaranteed you'll never see it again! You may have read this book and understood it, but when you re-read it you'll understand certain aspects you missed the first time. You also need to re-read it – or at least certain chapters – if you feel any doubt or any of the brainwashing creeping back in. Alternatively, get hold of a re-tuning Juice Master CD (see page 309) and play it in your car or use the hypnotherapy part of it to send you to sleep at night.

Even if you feel fantastic and don't feel you need a re-tune, it's still good to refresh your memory and keep this stuff clear in your mind. Remember you can't see brainwashing creeping back in, you only know it as a thought or doubt at some point in the future. Should you get them – re-tune and clear your mind. It is good to keep this stuff clear in your mind to counter the thousands of false ads and pieces of misinformation we see and hear daily. The more you hear, read and live this stuff the more it becomes your life. Whatever you focus on becomes real to you, so it's good to re-fresh your memory and keep focused.

One of the best ways to re-tune is to totally immerse yourself for a day in the subject. I don't mean sit indoors trying to re-tune and focus,

I mean giving yourself a real mental pick-me-up with a Juice Master seminar every now and then (maybe once every six months). With a book or even a CD you can easily get distracted or interrupted, but in a seminar you get to focus on the subject in hand for 6–7 hours.

I have quite a few clients who attend a seminar a couple of times a year simply for a re-tune and to stay well and truly juiced. They don't mind investing time and money to boost their batteries. It always seems odd to me that if the exhaust goes on your car, you find the time and the money to fix it – yet so many people think twice about investing in the single most important vehicle they will ever have the good fortune to own. Your mind needs investment; if you don't invest the batteries will wear down and someone else will charge them full of rubbish. The clients who come back every six months do so because it's effective. As one client puts it, (yes hello Gary T) 'It's like charging your mental batteries'. Of all the ways you can re-tune, it is also the most fun! And fun works for me. The one day ultimate health seminars are designed to be fun, moving and life-changing. There's not only the info in this book, there's also music, dancing and games such as WHO WANTS TO BE A SLIMIONAIRE?! You get to experience and do 'The Best Exercise Programme In The World', and shatter your 'people phobia'. You also get the chance to see juicing in action and sample some.

I realize this sounds a bit like an ad, but I am so passionate about what I do that I want your success to be forever – and I know how important it is to re-tune for that to be a reality. You don't have to come to a seminar, you can just immerse yourself in the book every now and then or just listen to the CD – whatever works for you. But please don't ignore this ingredient – it's very, very important. Your health and the way you feel both physically and mentally on a daily basis is the single most important thing in the world and I will do and say everything in my power to make certain you not only get to where you want to go, but that you stay there. And I want to make certain that you do whatever is necessary to…

Avoid the war

I want you to imagine that there is a war going on where two out of three people die and even those who survive are often very ill or disabled due to the enemy's sustained attack. Now I want you to imagine that you *have* to go. Every man and woman has been called up and you too are on the list. However, there is a way to get a reprieve, a way to avoid this horrific war: you have to make some fresh beautiful-tasting juice every day, eat some water-rich salad, go out and play, and get a re-tune every now and then.

What do you do?
NOT DIFFICULT TO ANSWER REALLY IS IT?

The truth is there really is a war going on and the NHS is desperately trying to deal with the casualties every day. The problem is they're so busy treating the wounded that they haven't the time to do anything about actually trying to *prevent* the war. It really doesn't matter how much money we throw at the NHS, it only goes on treating the casualties. This of course is very necessary. The problem, however, will only ease when we all do our bit to HELP PREVENT THE WAR. Every time someone breaks free from the food trap they are doing their bit. You can only be a casualty of war if you are there – by avoiding the war you are, in all likelihood, avoiding the white building with the red cross on it!

There are 8.3 million cases of *recognised* food poisoning reported each year in the UK alone. There are 31,000 deaths directly attributed to obesity, with a cost to the NHS of £2.6bn. I could go on like this forever but the point is the death toll because of 'food' is more than all drugs on the planet COMBINED, and the true cost to the NHS for treating all drug food and drink related diseases is tens of £billions. The war is raging, but you now can use your ticket to avoid it.

If ever I feel tired and can't be bothered to juice, I just think about the war and ask myself how much hassle is it really. As far as I'm concerned it's a lot easier to spend 15 minutes making juice than it is to deal with cancer, heart disease, strokes or God knows what kind of other horrific disease. It's amazing how just that thought alone can get you juicing happily in no time. By keeping your mind free of all the rubbish and flooding it with some mental juice whenever you can, you can achieve optimum health and live your *one and only* life in a light, slim, sexy, energy-driven body.

So keep flooding your body with physical juice, keep flooding your mind with mental juice, take the time to *enjoy* the flight and send me a postcard. I get a real kick every time I hear of the changes people have made because of the information in this book. I would love to hear from you and who knows, I just might see you for some dancing and juicing and a game of 'who wants to be a slimionaire' at some point in the future.

I will leave you with one final thought. When George Burns turned 87 years of age he sent out invitations to all of his friends to come to his 100th birthday party. He hated letting people down and knew by handing out the invites he just had to show up on the day – and of course he did. Enjoy today and always have something to look forward to – it keeps you alive in every way.

Smile, design your own life and enjoy the journey.

L.I.F.E.
Live In Fearless Excitement

Stay Juiced!

43
JM's Combining Tips

Remember – combining is simply a *tool* to better health, it is not an absolute *rule* to be adhered to at all times. This is, after all, nutrition for the real world! The body *can* deal with any combination of food we put in, but, we must remember, often at tremendous cost to our health and longevity. There is no question that the body copes much, much better when it has fewer combinations of 'man-made' foods to deal with. Ideally, you should make a point of only having one 'JM junk' food at each meal, and combining it with water-rich, nutrient-packed live foods.

Timing and combining rules for fruit

Fruit should be eaten *ideally* on an empty stomach, this is why I highly recommend it first thing in the morning – you can be sure the stomach is empty then. I also recommend fruit *before* a meal as opposed to after it. Having said that though, there are many fruits which contain enzymes that help to digest certain foods. Pineapple, lemons, oranges, pears, grapefruits, apricots, papayas, kiwis, peaches and blueberries for example all help to digest protein. Apple, for instance, has always been eaten with pork to aid digestion. Bananas, mango, raisins and dates aid the digestion of carbs. So a banana sandwich, or banana on cereal would go. Common sense seems to point to the juicy fruits going well with the proteins and the sugary, starchy fruits helping out the carbs.

There is one main rule with fruit. Unless you eat it at the same time or immediately after a meal of concentrated foods, wait until your stomach is empty again before eating it. This is because if you wait a while after a cooked meal to eat fruit, the other foods will have dropped to the lower part of the stomach and you risk indigestion and the fruit simply sitting and fermenting.

COMBINING

Which foods combine well?
Protein with a *small* portion of carbohydrate and loads of salad,
     veggies and/or veggie juice – YES
Carbohydrate with a *small* portion of protein plus salad,
     veggies and/or veggie juice – YES
Equal portions of *hard-to-digest* protein and carbohydrate at same
     time – NO (where possible – be flexible)
Equal *small* portions of *easy-to-digest* protein, natural fats and whole
     carbs – YES

The difference if you combine your foods well is a massive 5–8 hours worth of valuable nerve energy. That's 5–8 hours of free energy to help the body repair and rid itself of excess waste (that's fat to you and me). For best results eat just one concentrated food at a time. The next best is two of the same kind. So whenever you eat some chicken or fish, have as much as you feel like – just makes sure you combine it with a big water-rich salad and or some steamed or stir-fried veg. To make life easy I have produced a Juice Master wall-chart, which illustrates the combining tips at a glance, along with a few mental tips to get you inspired every day (see page 309).

RULES FOR MAKING JUICES

When it comes to juices there is, in fact, only one rule: vegetable and fruit juices don't mix that well together. The one exception to this is apple juice. Having said that if you were to have an *orange* and carrot juice it will still be of benefit, but the general rule is not to mix your fruit and veg juice, except apple.

In order to make sure that your veg juices taste wonderful every time here's a JM tip. Make sure that $1/2$ to $3/4$ of your veg juice is made up of either apple, carrot or tomato juice or a combination of these. Personally I'm not a fan of tomato juice so I either have a carrot juice base or a mixture of carrot and apple (commonly known as crapple – bad name I know). In fact virtually every veg juice I make has a crapple base. You will understand why if you try and do a veg juice without it: I once had leek, spinach and celery – it was nearly enough to put me off for life. So other than getting the base right and remembering that as a rule most fruit juices and veg juices don't mix very well together, you really are free to concoct your very own juice magic!

This is of course all very well and good, but at this stage you probably haven't got a juicer and if you do own one, in all likelihood it's not only gathering dust but the chances are it's not a patch on the one I recommend.

44

Equipment

THE BEST JUICING MACHINE IN THE WORLD
At the moment

I say 'at the moment' because, like everything, juicers can always be improved upon. They are not perfect – yet. I have a design for what I believe would be the best juicing machine in the world – so if there are any manufacturing companies looking to invest in The Juice Master juice extractor, let me know and we'll build it. Meanwhile, what exactly is the best juicing machine in the world? Well, to qualify for that title it has to be the easiest to use, easiest to clean and involve the least hassle and time. It also needs to be good value and be able to make loads of juice without you having to take it apart and clean it every two minutes. And, very important this, it has to have a large chute so you don't have to muck about chopping everything into a billion different pieces. And it goes without saying that it has to look good, have a good motor and be able to juice both fruit and veg with ease. That is the kind of machine that gets the JM seal of approval and title of The Best Juicing Machine In The World. And at the moment there is only one machine to my knowledge that fits the bill, ladies and gentlemen I give you –

THE JUICE MASTER PLUS
By Moulinex

Well, I don't actually give you – you have to invest – but what an investment this little space-age looking machine is. What's more, compared to its much lesser rivals in the starter juicer market, it's an absolute bargain.

Do you remember this?

'Moulinex Makes Things Simple And That Includes The Price'

Yes, perhaps another 'bell', but this one's right on the button. The Juice Master Plus is one of Moulinex's newest models and, like all of their juicing range, the design, motor and juicing capabilities are simply the best *by far* in the starter juicer market. I still have no idea how they put together such an incredible machine for so little money. You can pick this baby up for just £49.99 and this even includes a copy of *The Juice Master's Ultimate Fast Food* book. This beauty has a 400-watt motor, 2 speeds for soft and hard fruits, a larger than usual feeder chamber and is available in graphite and white. If I sound pretty impressed by this machine, it's because I am. My first ever juicer was the Moulinex 753P1, this machine just went on and on and on – the motor just didn't burn out (unusual for a starter machine). This is why I was keen to test this new model, and it didn't disappoint. It has a larger 'pulp' container than the 753P1 and it has an even better and more powerful motor. In my humble Juice Master opinion you just won't find a better starter juicer on the market and at that price it will be the best buy in your kitchen.

If you find after a while that your juicing needs become even greater, look out for The Juice Master Pro – coming Spring 2005.

For speed purposes in the morning it's also a great idea to get yourself a good citrus juicer. This enables you to make some orange juice without having to peel them. All you do is cut them in half and pull down on the lever or squeeze them onto the electric spinny thing (well I don't know what you call it!). You can then use this juice to add liquid to your blender full of soft fruits. This saves time on peeling and cleaning as it takes seconds to clean a citrus juicer and blender. You can then make your veg juice with your main juicer.

THE CHAMPION OF CHAMPIONS

There are a couple of other juicers which I highly recommend – the Champion (very aptly named) and the Green Star. These machines retail at £349 and £399 respectively and are the gold standards of the juicing world – strictly for the serious juicer. To many, they're not cheap, but think how much the average nutrient-destroying cooker is! These machines extract the juice in a completely different way to the normal juicers; crushing the produce at low speed, which leaves all the essential enzymes, vitamins and antioxidants intact. This 'masticating' action also leaves the pulp very dry – meaning more juice, less waste and so money saved. You can also make delicious pure fruit ice-creams and sorbets, smooth nut butter and homogenized baby food. The downside to the Green Star is it struggles with soft fruits and was really specifically designed for veggies, where it performs magnificently, managing to even juice wheatgrass. The Champion, however, is much more versatile, juicing all fruits with ease, is cheaper and comes with a massive 5-year guarantee. To be fair, it's hard to choose between the two, but one thing's for sure, the smooth creamy vegetable juice you get from these machines is unsurpassed and the investment in your health - priceless. For most people, though, the Juice Master Plus and a decent blender are more than sufficient.

And when it comes to blenders our friends at Moulinex have once again come up trumps – this time with the Juice Master's Chicago smoothie maker. It has a glass jug, ice crusher and makes smoothies beautifully. The one thing which is impressive is again its amazing value and versatility. The motor is built to last and it blends nuts, ices and frozen fruits with ease. There are of course many blenders on the market, from the starter hand-held ones, which are fine (like the Moulinex Turbo Mix at just £11.99), to ones that come as part of a food processor, and glass jug ones. Have a look around to see what meets your budget and needs.

A blender really is your best friend in the morning – if you are in a hurry, you can just put some soft fruits in, add some ice, blend and go. It is also the only way to add fruits like bananas to your juice to make a smoothie. Whatever you do DON'T TRY TO JUICE A BANANA – it's a waste of time, effort and money, Bananas always go in the blender along with so many other soft fruits – and ice to cool it down. So where can I get my hands on these machines, Mr Juice Master? If you are on the world wide web, simply look at our website, if not simply call our juicy hotline number (details at back).

So what else will I need?

A good chopping knife and a large chopping board. These two items are also essential for regular juicing and salad making. The last thing you need is a blunt knife slowing you down. A big chopping board is also important. You will be using it a lot for salads, stir-fried veg and cutting things for juices. So invest once and then it's done.

So is that it, can I get cracking now?

Don't see why not. To help you get started I've included some Juice Master recipes. These are some of my favourites – there's nothing to stop you creating some of your own, so be flexible and experiment. Happy juicing.

45

Recipes

LET'S GET FRUITY

THE JACK 'SUN' FIVE

A little nutty, but makes your body move and makes you feel soooooo good inside – it's easy as 1, 2, 3 doh, ray me.

You will need
- 2 peaches
- Handful of ice
- Small handful of almonds
- Handful of frozen berries (your choice – try black forest fruits)
- $^1/_2$ medium pineapple
- 4 oranges
- $^1/_4$ grapefruit

What you do with it
Put peaches in blender (yes take out stone first or you will have no blender left!) and add the ice, nuts and berries. Juice the pineapple, oranges and grapefruit and pour into the other ingredients in the blender. Blend until smooth and creamy, then drink and let your cells sing.

THE BERRY MAGUIRE

'Show me the honey'

You will need
- 1 good handful of frozen blackberries
- 1 good handful of fresh strawberries
  (replace with frozen raspberries if necessary)
- $1^1/_2$ mugs of cranberry or orange juice
- $^1/_2$ mug of mineral water
- Small handful of ice
- 1 heaped teaspoon of organic honey (raw if possible)

What you do with it

Put the whole lot in your blender and blend until smooth – drink and enjoy.

Note: Use your common sense when it comes to amounts. If what I list makes too much or too little juice for your needs, just change the amounts. All the recipes are just rough guidelines, as always be flexible.

THE CARIBBEAN DREAM

This is the Rolls-Royce of smoothies – it's pure sunshine for your cells. It's a real treat but soooooo worth it.

You will need
- 1 coconut
- $^1/_4$–$^1/_2$ of medium-sized mango
- Half a papaya
- 1 banana
- A handful of ice (or small cup of cold mineral water)
- 1 medium pineapple
- 3–4 oranges or $^1/_2$ grapefruit (your choice)

What you do with it

Using a bottle opener, drill a hole in one of the three dimples on the coconut and pour the fresh coconut milk into the blender. Add mango chunks, papaya, banana and ice or water. Juice the pineapple and oranges or grapefruit. Pour the juice into the blender and blend until smooth for heaven in a glass.

Note: The white flesh of the coconut can then be eaten with it if you wish (although it's a real bugger to get it out I can tell ya).

SPRING BREAK-FAST

A juice to help break your fast with a touch of spring.

You will need

- 4 oranges
- $1/_2$ pink grapefruit
- Spring water with bubbles (I recommend Perrier)
- 5 ice cubes

What you do with it

Juice the oranges and grapefruit. Pour into blender, add a glass of spring water and the ice. Blend, pour, drink and let the joys of spring furnish every cell in your body.

THE MS LEWINSKY

A high protein drink – with nuts of course!

Nothing goes down as good as this, but watch your clothes – it could stain.

You will need (a good lawyer, sorry I mean...)

- 2 plums (I know)
- 1 banana (stop it!)
- 1 coconut (it gets worse trust me)

🍓 Handful of nuts (make that ¹/₂ handful almonds)
🍓 A good pear (well 4 of the conference variety)
🍓 Ice, ice, baby

What you do with it

Seed the plums and put in the blender with the banana and almonds. Using a corkscrew, drill a hole in one of the three dimples in the coconut and pour the milk into the blender. Juice the pears (take the stems off first) and add to blender. Blend all the ingredients until smooth, drink and enjoy.

US ELECTION SPECIAL 2000

Have you the 'Gore' to try this one?

You will need

🍓 4 peaches
🍓 4 Florida oranges
🍓 ¹/₂ a Florida grapefruit
🍓 6 ice cubes

What you do with it

Stone peaches and place in blender. Take them out and count them again just to make sure you have the correct number. Put back in and immediately seek an injunction to prevent them being counted again. Once the injunction has been turned down, count them again and place back in blender. Now count oranges until you are blue in the face and then take skin off – in other words reject the ap-*peel* (sorry – yes I know that was bad). Do the same with the grapefruit. Juice oranges, grapefruit and pour into blender. Add ice, blend, pour, drink and enjoy.

TIME TO 'VEG OUT'

CRAPPLE JUICE

This is made up of carrot and apple and is the base that I use for virtually all my vegetable juices. The reason for this is taste. Have you ever tried a spinach and beetroot juice by itself? How about leek? Well trust me, they take a lot of getting used to and I don't want you to be put off veg juice as it's very important in building up your vitamin and mineral bank account. On that note – DON'T JUICE GARLIC. If you do, every juice you make for a week afterwards reeks of the stuff.

I always make sure that at least 50–75 per cent of my veg juice is made up of crapple juice (if you prefer you could use a carrot or tomato juice base – this is just my favourite). You then add whatever you like on top: celery, spinach, beetroot, cucumber, cabbage, etc.

To make about 1 pint of crapple juice, you'll need 1kg of carrots and around four apples. Simply juice the lot and enjoy as it is or use as a base. If you are using crapple as a base remember that the added veg should make up about one third of the whole juice (the usual amount needed in this case is about 500g carrots to 2–3 apples).

THE IRON LADY

No 'tis not a Mrs Thatcher – we're talking beneficial iron here (only joking).

You will need
Some carrots and apples (crapple base). Enough to make 50–75% of overall content of juice.

- Piece of broccoli
- Handful of spinach
- Handful of kale

What you do with it
Simply juice the lot, pour and enjoy.

You can use organically grown green stuff, but unless you own something like a 'Green Life' juicer, there is a lot of waste. I do, however, tend to use organic carrots and apples for the base, even if I'm using my Breville.

THE DY'SUN'

Picks up rubbish from your blood and cleans out your colon – all without the need for a bag!

You will need

Apple and carrot base

- 1 palm-sized raw beetroot
- 2 sticks of celery
- $^1/_2$ medium cucumber
- Good handful of spinach

What you do with it

Juice the lot, stir, pour and enjoy.

This is much easier to get right first time than the real 'Dyson'. It took the incredible Mr Dyson over 4000 attempts to get it right – and people say he was lucky!

HAWNY JUICE

No – it doesn't make you feel horny. It's named after the beautiful Goldie Hawn. This juice is said to be one of the reasons why she stays looking so damn good. She is a huge juicing fan and this is one of her faves.

You will need

- 4 large carrots
- $^1/_2$ cucumber
- 3 sticks of celery

What you do with it

Juice the lot, stir and pour the liquid goldie into your cells

---

BROCCOLI SPEARS

Oh baby, baby – a juice 'virgin' on the divine.

What you need

'Crapple' base (apple and carrot)

- 2 big handfuls of broccoli (including spears)
- $1/_4$ of a large cucumber (for that clean, fresh-faced look)

What you do with it

Simply juice the lot and let your system feel 'Stronger' (that's a Britney song in case you didn't know) whilst your cells are singing 'Hit me baby one more time'.

As with all juices/smoothies make adjustments with quantities depending on amount of juice required.

THE NICK LEESON

Designed to totally clean you out! Perhaps this is the only time it's worth investing in a 'Nick Leeson' – this one actually helps to replenish your bank account (of the enzyme kind at least)!

You will need

- 10 carrots
- 1 raw beetroot
- $1/_2$ cucumber
- 1 stick celery
- 2 large handfuls of spinach
- 1 handful of broccoli
- $1/_4$ lemon
- $1/_4$ lime

What you do with it

Top and tail carrots and peel lemon and lime. Juice everything and if warm, place in blender with a little ice. Pour, drink and know that every time you have a 'Nick Leeson' you have added to your bank account of pure life force. Remember, if you don't invest the system will go into receivership and BOOM – show's over!

GINGER ROGERS AND FRED A PEAR

A truly unbelievable combination.

You will need
- ½ lemon
- 2 tomatoes
- 5 carrots
- ¼ inch cube of ginger
- 3 apples
- ½ ripe avocado pear (make sure there is a little give as you squeeze)

What you do with it

Juice lemon, tomatoes, carrots, apples and ginger. Put avocado pear into blender then add the juice. Blend until creamy and let the nutrients dance with your cells!

THE ULTIMATE JUICE MASTER SALAD

You can use just about any fruit, veg, fish or meat to make a salad, but here is my ultimate main course salad.

You will need
- Young leaf spinach, bag of mixed salad leaves (whichever you prefer),
- tomatoes (whichever you prefer – cherry, plum, etc.), red onion, red pepper,
- orange pepper, yellow pepper, cucumber, red cabbage, white cabbage,
- 1 carrot, alfalfa sprouts, avocados (as many as you like)
- Dressing: 1 teaspoon olive oil, 2 capfuls balsamic vinegar (white if possible) and juice of one lemon.

What you do with it

Tear baby spinach into small pieces and place in a large salad bowl along with the bag of salad leaves. Cut and add tomatoes, onion, peppers, and cucumber (as thick or thin as you like). Grate some cabbage and all the carrot, then add to bowl along with the alfalfa sprouts. Mix the dressing ingredients together, add to the bowl and give it all a good mix. Cut the avocados into strips and place around side of bowl, sprinkle more lemon juice over the avocados.

Eat as it is, stuff inside warm pitta bread or have it with chicken, tuna, fish, egg or combination of all – have it your way. You can, of course, add whatever you like to this including, pineapple, mango, walnuts and grated apple. Experiment and enjoy.

JUICE MASTER'S GUACAMOLE

This is my favourite dip and it's not only scrumptious, it's good for you.

You will need
- 6 medium ripe avocados
- Juice of 2 lemons
- 1 clove of garlic
- 2 tomatoes
- 1 small onion (red or white)
- Handful of chives
- 2 small green chillies (these are optional – if you do use them remember to leave out the seeds, unless you like to blow your head off)

What you do with it

Peel and seed the avocados and put in the blender with the lemon juice. Put garlic through garlic press and add to blender. Make sure you push the avocado well into the blender with a spoon. Blend until creamy (you may have to stop and start blender a few times and keep moving ingredients around). Finely chop the tomatoes, onion, chives and chillies. Spoon out the creamy avocado dip from the blender and place in bowl. Add the chopped ingredients and mix together. Serve with just about anything and enjoy.

46
Q & A

 As I will be drinking so much liquid with my juices, do I need to drink water?

Water is an essential part of all life on the planet – without it we would all soon perish. However, this does not mean you need to drown your body with gallons of the stuff. Obviously you should drink water according to your thirst, but be aware that most of the time we don't actually realize we are becoming dehydrated. I therefore recommend that in addition to your juices, salads and fruits, that you help your body to cleanse itself and stay hydrated by drinking 2 litres of water every day. If you're working out or in high sun then clearly more – just use your common sense.

What is the difference between a juice and a smoothie?

A smoothie is a combination of whole soft fruits and either milk, yogurt, or fruit juice mixed together in a blender. Obviously I skip the white glue stuff and use ice, fruit juice and some water with added soft fruits. If you're in a real hurry you can add organic soya milk once in a while, although it doesn't taste as good. The reason for adding juice is so that the mixture isn't too thick. This is the biggest mistake people make when making smoothies – they tend to just stick whole fruits into a blender and whisk them up. If you do this it's too thick, so add some liquid. You can deliberately make it thick and eat it like an ice cream. Just put a load of frozen fruits into a blender add a little ice – eat and enjoy. I nearly always have smoothies when it comes to fruit and always have just the juice when it comes to veg.

Is yogurt just as bad as milk?

Yes and no really, it all depends on the particular kind of yogurt. Most yogurts are heavily processed and contain quite a bit of sugar – they are also nutritionally dead. If you want yogurt every now and then, choose the 'live' versions. Live yogurt has what's called 'friendly bacteria' present and this stuff can actually be very good for you. But as with anything which comes from the inside of an animal – every now and then is fine, but not all the time.

Are there different kinds of milk I can have?

Yes. There are many different kinds of milk on the market that are much, much better than cow's milk. Although you can buy milks such as soya and rice, you can easily make your own in seconds using your blender. If you put a couple of bananas in a blender and add some ice and water, you can blend them all to make banana milk. Add some almond nuts and you've got banana and almond milk. If you do buy soya milk it's worth buying the unsweetened organic version as a lot of soya is genetically modified. Having said all of that, you will find that most of the time you won't need a replacement for milk, as you will be free from the foods that you used to add milk to. The only time I use soya milk or the home-made versions is when I choose to have some muesli for lunch or 'flexi breakfast' at times. Even then I only use milk if I haven't the time to juice some apples. Fresh apple juice poured over muesli is simply scrumptious. Don't knock it till you've tried it. One more thing – avoid all powdered milks.

You've talked about how wonderful mother's milk is for babies, but I can't breast feed. What should I feed my baby?

I realize there will be many women reading this book who, for whatever reason, cannot breast feed. If you are wondering what the hell you can feed your baby, please remember that a baby has the correct enzymes to break down milk – it's only adults who have the problem. In fact it is essential, *an absolute must* that babies get milk of some kind. If you want the nearest thing possible to mother's milk then goat's milk, organic carrot juice and water is the best you can get. A goat has one stomach like us so the baby can not only deal with this type of milk much easier than cows, but it thrives on it.

Is it possible to live on nothing but fruit, veg and juices?

Yes indeed, as long as you throw in a few nuts and seeds for good measure. It is more than possible and yes you would be extremely healthy, but having *nothing* but raw food 24/7– well it's not for me. I once had nothing but freshly extracted fruit and veg juices for three months and trust me, that's a looooong time to go on just juices. The only reason I did it was to try and clear my skin of psoriasis. I lost far too much weight to the point where I made Ally McBeal look fat! You cannot, nor should not, live on juice alone – **you need fibre**. The maximum time you should have a juice clearout for is 5–7 days. I often have days where I eat nothing but raw foods and drink fresh juices – in fact my intake even when I'm eating cooked foods on a particular day tends to be 70–80 per cent natural fast food. But I am not obsessive and I'm incredibly flexible – it depends on where I am or who I'm with. If you want to eat nothing but fruit, veg, nuts and seeds and you are perfectly happy doing it then brilliant – it will serve you more than well. But as far as I'm concerned, it is just too restrictive in today's world, especially when we have dinner parties and especially when there is simply no need to. The body was designed to deal with a certain amount of just about anything – so eat, relax and enjoy!

What about eggs?

Umm – I guess if we really thought about what an egg is, we'd probably never go near them. In terms of health, eggs are not that good. They are, however, a JM junk food and not a drug food, which means if you want some boiled eggs on your salad, or the *occasional* omelette, feel free. I recommend no more than about 3–4 eggs a week and strongly recommend leaving them out of the frying pan. Once again 'organic' applies in this case as, trust me, the things I could tell you about eggs produced from battery hens could fill another book.

What about dried fruit?

Dried fruits are not only delicious, but are very good for you – if used in moderation. My favourite is dried mango – it's simply orgasmic. Do check the label though, as many of those on sale contain sulphur dioxide, which is caustic to the stomach. As always, go for the natural, nothing-added variety. The general rule is if they look too bright and cheery there's probably some chemical involved somewhere.

Note: dried fruits are high in sugar and, although natural, they are very concentrated so please use sparingly. If diabetic or hypoglycaemic – leave well alone.

Fruit is also high in sugar so won't it cause the same problems as white sugar?

NO, NO, NO, NO, NO, NO! Sorry for the outburst, but since the 'eat nothing but fat and protein diet' I know several people who are convinced that fruit sugar causes the same problems as the white refined kind and so they eat fried eggs, bacon and sausages instead of a piece of fruit. For their purposes, as well as yours, I want to make this next point very clear. *There is a massive difference between the sugar you find in fresh fruit and the white refined drug variety.* The sugar you find in fruit has many different elements to it. It is a whole food, contains bundles of life-giving nutrients and is high in water, which helps to transport the goodness to the cells and flush out the waste. White refined sugars and carbs contain *nothing* of any value to the body – they are totally empty foods. I will repeat that the only time fruit can be a problem is if you gulp down a pint of smoothie in a very short amount of time. Once again if you are diabetic – either dilute your juice with half mineral water, or just eat the fruit and juice your vegetables.

This juicing thing sounds a bit of a hassle, do I have to buy a juicer and juice every day for this to be a success?

No you don't. That may sound a bit strange coming from the JUICE MASTER and all, but I want to make it clear that juicing is meant to be used as a *tool* – a catalyst to get you to the land of the slim and healthy. Whilst I wholeheartedly believe in juicing as perhaps the best way possible to get nutrients into an already battered and clogged system, and as an incredible aid help flush out waste, I'm not so arrogant to say it's the only way. If you prefer to *eat* all your fruit and are quite happy *eating* plenty of steamed, lightly cooked or raw vegetables EVERY DAY then feel free to do so. Just make certain that at least 70 per cent of what you eat is live natural food, with fish, white lean meat, whole grains and tiny amounts of dairy making up the remaining 30 per cent. However, I obviously strongly advise using juicing as a tool for your health – especially while you are on the journey to wellness and vibrancy. It's like going *fast track* as opposed to economy! Once you have arrived in the land of slim and healthy and are 'maintaining' then you may find you are using your juicer slightly less and eating raw more. As with everything – use your common sense.

In the recipes you don't mention how much juice each one will make – is there a reason for this?

Yes, I have done this for three reasons. Firstly, it all depends on which juicer you use. They vary, so it's no good me stating that if you juice 500g of carrots you will get ½ a pint as your machine could yield less or more. Secondly, the age and origin of the fruit or veg will also play its part in the amount of juice they contain: not all carrots, even if they're the same size and they're juiced in the same machine, will yield the same amount of juice. Thirdly, and perhaps most importantly, I want to get away from the usual juice recipe books that don't allow for flexibility or your own imagination. Having said all that, each recipe in this book will give you very roughly 1–1½ pints of juice, but the best way to find out how much each one will make is to make it and see. If you find it makes too much for your requirements, simply adjust amounts accordingly. Trust me, as long as you follow the JM combining tips and basic rules/guidelines for juice (pages 282–3) you can experiment till your heart's content and become a master of the juice yourself.

When looking for 'whole' meal/grain breads and carbs, which ones are okay?

Well the best of the best for health are unleavened breads that contain no flour, yeast, sugars or oils, but still have all the fibre and germ of the whole grain. These breads are made from sprouted grains such as spelt, millet, flax, oats, kamut and quinoa (you can find these at some supermarkets and all good health stores).

Although these are the best, I can almost guarantee, unless you have a real yeast and wheat problem, they will not be the ones you choose all the time. The best choice, I believe, is wholemeal pitta bread. You can warm them slightly in the oven, open them up and stuff them full of water-rich, nutrient-packed salad. Rye bread is also pretty good: toast two slices, spread on loads of creamy avocado and pack out with a water-rich salad. Other acceptable complex carbs are as follows (but please remember these should make up no more than about 20–25 per cent of your total food intake and should ideally be consumed with plenty of water-rich JM fast food): whole rolled oats, whole-wheat pastas, whole-wheat tortillas, brown rice (not instant), stone ground whole-wheat flour, whole-grain crackers, dark rye crackers, stone ground whole-wheat bagels, stone ground whole-wheat breads, wholemeal breads, whole-wheat croutons.
So, quite a feast!

How much weight can I expect to lose in what time frame?

One of the key instructions is not to be a weight watcher, not to play the 'I'll be happy when' game, but if you want to know how long it's going to take before you personally lose your **excess** weight, here is a rough idea. The average person I see, who follows the physical and mental ultimate health recipe, drops about 6–14lb in weight in the first month and then an average of 2lb a week thereafter. But please understand there are no hard and fast rules here, there are many factors to consider. If you are already slim, or only have a few pounds to lose, then clearly you are not going to lose more weight than is healthy following this programme. It's only if you do an 'Ally McBeal' that you'll end up unnaturally thin. Remember, nature's idea of perfect shape and what the media often portrays can be worlds apart. I once had a young lady phone me and say, 'I'm following everything you said but after the first month I stopped losing weight'. It turned out she was already just 8st (104lbs): for her height it sounded about right, maybe even a little too thin – one thing's for sure, she wasn't fat! It would take a completely unnatural diet for her to get to what she believes is an ideal weight. Remember, it may be 'ideal' for fashion editors and models but not for those of us who live in the real world.

Your body may already be *its* ideal weight and shape, but *you* are still fighting to achieve what you believe is the 'ideal look'. It's a battle you are bound to lose and why start it in the first place? I will never be a strapping six footer with a body like Russell Crowe – no matter what the hell I eat – and you may never look like Nicole Kidman, but so what. As long as we are feeling good, looking good, living (as opposed to simply surviving) and are truly free in every sense of the word then we should be grateful for the body we do have, give thanks for our health and rejoice at being alive.

Of course many people reading this book will be overweight and trying to get slimmer. Often people with quite a bit of weight to lose find that they drop a bit of weight and then plateau for while, to the point where it seems they are 'stuck'. This happens for a good reason. The body does things at its own speed – what's most important to you may well not be what's most important for the wellness of the whole body. There is a good chance that over the years you have damaged tissues or organs and you may also have asthma, arthritis, IBS, or other problems. Now as far as your body is concerned rectifying damage and disease and making you well again might be far more important to it at times than dropping a few pounds. So what usually happens is you drop some weight and then seemingly nothing happens for a short time, then you drop some more and so it goes. As long as you are supplying your body with nutrients and oxygen, and keeping it free from the majority of toxic food products, you can be guaranteed that even if nothing appears to be happening, it is. So trust me, the body will drop excess weight when *it* feels it's safe to do so, just don't sit around waiting. If you cut your finger you get on with your life and let your body do what it needs to do to repair it – you certainly don't sit there staring at it waiting for it to get better do you? So don't do the same here. Remember – do it right once and you will never have a weight problem again. If you still feel the weight not shifting do the following –

1. Have a 2-day pure water and lemon cleanse.
2. Eat your fruit and drink your veg.
3. Cut out all man-made carbohydrates for just two weeks.

Sometimes the pancreas is so badly damaged and the system so clogged that even the good stuff cannot get through, and even the most modest amounts of carbohydrates can cause an over-secretion of insulin, and we know by now that insulin is THE FAT PRODUCING HORMONE. So, if you are willing, for just two days, have at least five litres of water with slices of lemon/lime in (hot water with lemon/lime is good too). Then go 2–4 weeks of just eating your fruit, drinking your veg and cutting out all man-made carbohydrates. If you still don't start to see the results after this I'll eat my shorts!

But I'm not overweight, I read this just to learn more about food. In fact I'm underweight, will this be dangerous for me?

No way. This way of eating, breathing, thinking and living is healthy for every single human being on the planet and if you are underweight you will not lose more weight on this programme – you will in all likelihood return to a natural, healthy weight.

What about salad dressings?

Glue-ridden, toxic dressings seem to be the order of the day, both in cookbooks and on TV cookery programmes. Avoid these and 'change your brand' of dressing to one which will serve you. I tend to just have a mix of balsamic vinegar, virgin olive oil and lemon juice. Also try a fresh lemon and lime dressing – it's simple but wonderful. Every now and then I will have a Caesar salad when out and yes I know Caesar dressing is far from the best, but once in a while is fine – remember, feel free.

Nuts!

Nuts to you too! Any nut which has been roasted and salted is not only 'lifeless' but very detrimental to the body and because of the white refined salt, also addictive. Natural nuts, on the other hand, are an excellent source of natural fats – Brazils, almonds, pistachios etc. are all superb.

I was on the loo a lot, had a few headaches and felt a bit, well, ill – is that normal on a *healthy* eating plan?

It can be, but please realize you're not ill – *you are getting better*. All that's happening is your body is having a good clean out. Don't worry – any discomfort you feel will soon subside and please bear in mind that any physical reactions you suffer are not because you've *stopped* eating and drinking the rubbish, but because you started in the first place. Your body is full of toxic waste and it needs to go somewhere, so if you do find yourself on the loo a lot during the first couple of weeks – GOOD. In no time at all you will be looking and feeling better than you have in years – happy cleaning!

Can I have the odd dip?

Yes, there is nothing wrong with having dips every now and then, but a dip means dip! Dips are meant to be there for you to dip into every now and then – not to have as your entire meal. Be careful with them; don't get into the habit of having pittas, dips and nothing else. High water content, 'live' nutrient based meals are the key to life-long success and if all you have after a hard day at work is dips and bread you will be consuming 0 per cent water-rich, live-nutrient packed food. *All* of the ready-made dips you buy are nutritionally *dead* – the enzymes were destroyed during processing. Most are also full of cow glue and chemicals. I am not saying don't have them, but please be aware they fall into the 20–30 per cent of non-natural food your body can easily deal with. Exceptions to cow glue dips are hummus, taramasalata and guacamole. The best are hummus and guacamole, both of which you can make yourself. I personally love home-made guacamole – it's creamy, tastes sensational, and is high in water and essential live nutrients. You can use it as a spread, dip, or add water and balsamic vinegar for beautiful salad dressing, or pour straight over jacket potatoes. And it's so easy to make – see JM's Guacamole in recipe section.

When it comes to quick pitta snacks, the key is to warm your pittas in the oven and stuff them full of high-water, nutrient-rich salad or stir-fried veg with perhaps some fresh pesto sauce. You can then use the dips for what they are – dips. Don't make them your whole meal, but it's more than okay to take the odd dip.

Is this stuff safe for my kids?

YES, YES, YES. It's eating and drinking the 'other stuff' that is not safe for your kids. I have seen many children in my seminars and I'd like to share a letter with you which I received from a young lady of 13 years of age called Patrina:

'Hi Jason...I just wanted to say a big big thank you for what you did for me, I really appreciate it. This new way of eating is great, I have loads more

energy. Thank you for sending me that letter it gave me more confidence that I can do it and thank you for recommending the juicer, it's great. I feel like I'm already on my way to Mauritius. Thanks again.'

Still not convinced?

'Just a quick note to let you know how you changed the life of a 16-year-old girl that attended your seminar. At the time she was around 13 stone and had been having weight problems since she was 10 or younger. You should see her now, she looks fantastic, beyond belief. I told her I was going to send you an email and she said "tell Jason he can send tickets for Mauritius any time now". I really wanted to say thank you very, very much.'

Helen

These are just a couple of the many children I have had the good fortune to coach to health over the years. Children not only thrive on this stuff – they love it. What they hate is being force-fed dead food, especially when it's a sunny afternoon and all they want to do is play. Many times as a child I would literally cry at the Sunday dinner table because I wasn't hungry for food but for oxygen and fun. Being force-fed is not only a nightmare for a child's sanity, but it is extremely unhealthy as you shouldn't eat when you're not hungry. It's made ten times worse when the food is totally lifeless and detrimental to the body.

I'm not picking on parents here, after all they are only doing what they have been taught is best, but if you do have children and want to also set them free – then don't worry on the health front. Most children will quite happily feast on fresh fruit all day given the choice and as for the fresh juices – they love them. Making juice in the morning becomes fun and kids will want to get involved with the process. As for the main meals, they will obviously be eating the same as you, so will be as healthy as pie.

Obviously you will not be able to change everything they eat but if you want a tip on how to make them change, here it is. Children are not stupid and, like us, hate being told what they can or cannot do.

Remember CAN'T is pure torture, and can't also creates a rebellious mind-set in children. Treat children like adults and explain to them exactly what these foods are doing and why you have chosen to be free from them. You will find that as long as you don't become a member of the 'food police' and keep telling them they can't, they will make the choice themselves – especially when you explain to them just how much better they will look and feel.

Are there any alternatives to salt?

Yes, health – that's a pretty good alternative to this stroke-inducing substance. Lemon juice is the best substitute for salt, as I have already mentioned: it may sound strange, but it really works. If you are going to have salt though, and if we deal with reality there will of course be odd times when you do, then buy the best coarsely grained sea salt you can get. When out in a restaurant use lemon juice where possible, but the little bit of salt you have on a meal out will not make that much difference.

If I do choose to stop eating meat, fish and all dairy products – where will I get my protein?

A very common question for the very few people who do decide to become vegan. In terms of sanity and flexibility I always advise that people don't avoid all animal products, but if you have made that choice, then I want to put your mind at rest when it comes to protein. Our protein is made of something called amino acids – there are 23 in all. The good news is that we already have 15 of them, the bad news is that it is essential to get the other eight from our diet. These eight are known as 'essential amino acids' because without them our health suffers. Despite what many of the 'experts' may say you can easily get all your essential amino acids through eating fruit, veg, grains and nuts – as long as you eat a variety of these foods. If you have a good varied diet you can be confident that you are getting all the protein you need. If in doubt, use your common sense – the largest and strongest land animal, the elephant, is a vegan!

THE JUICE MASTER'S PAGE

For information on the Juice Master's videos, books, CDs, tapes, up-and-coming Slim 4 Life seminars, Stop Smoking in 2 Hrs Guaranteed CD programme, Quit Alcohol programme, private sessions – plus anything else you need to know

Call the Juice Master Hotline on:
0845 1 30 28 29
(Please note this will cost you the price of a local call wherever you are in the UK.)
Website: www.thejuicemaster.com
Email: info@thejuicemaster.com
Post: Juicy Towers, 22 Moseley Gate, Birmingham, B13 8JJ

For information on where to buy the juicing machines/blenders, etc., mentioned in this book, please go to the main website (www.thejuicemaster.com) or phone the Juice Master hotline.